FRCS (Oral & Maxillofacial Surgery) Part 2

100 Clinical Cases

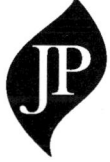

FRCS (Oral & Maxillofacial Surgery) Part 2

100 Clinical Cases

Johno Breeze PhD FRCS FDS
Consultant Oral and Maxillofacial Surgeon,
University Hospitals Birmingham, UK

Ross Elledge BChD(Hons) MBChB(Hons)
MMEd MFDSRCPS(Glasg) FRCS (OMFS)
Consultant Oral and Maxillofacial Surgeon,
University Hospitals Birmingham, UK

Rhodri Williams FDS MBChB FRCS(OMFS)
Consultant Oral and Maxillofacial Surgeon,
University Hospitals Birmingham, UK

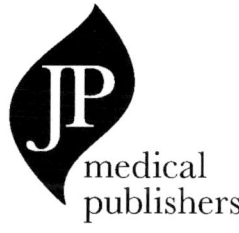

JP medical publishers

London • New Delhi

© 2020 Jaypee Brothers Medical Publishers
Published by Jaypee Brothers Medical Publishers,
4838/24 Ansari Road, New Delhi, India

Tel: +91 (011) 43574357   Fax: +91 (011)43574390

Email: info@jpmedpub.com, jaypee@jaypeebrothers.com
Web: www.jpmedpub.com, www.jaypeebrothers.com

JPM is the imprint of Jaypee Brothers Medical Publishers.

The rights of Johno Breeze, Ross Elledge and Rhodri Williams to be identified as editors of this work have been asserted by them in accordance with the Copyright, Designs and Patents Act 1988.

All rights reserved. No part of this publication may be reproduced, stored or transmitted in any form or by any means, electronic, mechanical, photocopying, recording or otherwise, except as permitted by the UK Copyright, Designs and Patents Act 1988, without the prior permission in writing of the publishers. Permissions may be sought directly from JP Medical Ltd at the address printed above.

All brand names and product names used in this book are trade names, service marks, trademarks or registered trademarks of their respective owners. The publisher is not associated with any product or vendor mentioned in this book.

Medical knowledge and practice change constantly. This book is designed to provide accurate, authoritative information about the subject matter in question. However, readers are advised to check the most current information available on procedures included and check information from the manufacturer of each product to be administered, to verify the recommended dose, formula, method and duration of administration, adverse effects and contraindications. It is the responsibility of the practitioner to take all appropriate safety precautions. Neither the publisher nor the authors assume any liability for any injury and/or damage to persons or property arising from or related to use of material in this book.

This book is sold on the understanding that the publisher is not engaged in providing professional medical services. If such advice or services are required, the services of a competent medical professional should be sought.

Every effort has been made where necessary to contact holders of copyright to obtain permission to reproduce copyright material. If any have been inadvertently overlooked, the publisher will be pleased to make the necessary arrangements at the first opportunity.

ISBN: 978-1-909836-83-9

British Library Cataloguing in Publication Data
A catalogue record for this book is available from the British Library

Library of Congress Cataloging in Publication Data
A catalog record for this book is available from the Library of Congress

Development Editor:	Harsha Madan
Editorial Assistant:	Keshav Kumar
Cover Design:	Seema Dogra

Preface

The FRCS(OMFS) examination can rightly be regarded as a key milestone in the life of any Oral and Maxillofacial Surgery trainee's life. Its completion signifies to the successful candi-date that the race to the completion of training and specialist registration is nearly won. The race is a marathon rather than a sprint however.

The breadth of knowledge required of candidates may appear daunting and insurmountable, but ultimately the exam should be regarded as the consolidation of the summative experience of training. Every clinic, every operating list, every ward round and every on call should have been leading up to this moment. Rather than "cramming", the good trainee will do what or he or she does every day with every patient.

The current work aims to help give an overview of what is required of trainees in approaching the FRCS(OMFS) and is the first of its kind in our specialty. The book aims to help trainees focus knowledge acquired in simulated patient encounters in the setting of the clinical exam. In making the leap to applying the theory, the trainee is directed through likely questions and pearls of current thinking that may distinguish the excellent trainee from the merely satisfactory one. At this level, there are no clear answers and understanding the evidence base may help you "argue" the case with an examiner holding conflicting views in areas where there is no right or wrong, at the limits of our knowledge. This is the higher order thinking expected in the exam.

Clearly the book is a touchstone and reference work, but throughout we aim to direct the reader to pivotal research papers and further reading for a deeper understanding in areas that he or she may wish to explore more thoroughly. Read this as a standalone work, use it as the springboard to wider reading or simulate the exam with colleagues. Above all, re-hearse saying the knowledge you already have out loud and have strength in your convic-tions about the greyer areas of the specialty. You are the next generation of surgeons.

Johno Breeze
Ross Elledge
Rhodri Williams
July 2019

Contents

Preface	v
Contributors	ix
About the examination	x
Abbreviations	xi
Acknowledgements	xv

Chapter 1	Dentoalveolar surgery	1
Chapter 2	Head and neck oncological surgery	25
Chapter 3	Orthognathic surgery	77
Chapter 4	Facial cutaneous surgery	127
Chapter 5	Facial trauma	155
Chapter 6	Salivary gland disease	195
Chapter 7	Oral pathology	217
Chapter 8	Temporomandibular joint surgery	261
Chapter 9	Craniofacial and paediatric surgery	291
Chapter 10	Cleft lip and palate surgery	313
Chapter 11	Facial aesthetic surgery	331

Contributors

Jagtar Dhanda PhD FRCS FDS
Consultant Oral and Maxillofacial Surgeon
University Hospitals Birmingham, UK

Steven Dover FDS RCS, FRCS
Consultant Oral and Maxillofacial Surgeon
University Hospitals Birmingham, UK

Demetrius Evriviades BSc MB ChB FRCSPlast PGDip
Consultant Plastic and Reconstructive Surgeon
University Hospitals Birmingham, UK

Jason Green MSc, FDSRCS, FRCS
Consultant Oral and Maxillofacial Surgeon
University Hospitals Birmingham, UK

Kevin McMillan MFD FRCS
Consultant Oral and Maxillofacial Surgeon
University Hospitals Birmingham, UK

Sat Parmar BMedSci, FDSRCS, FRCS
Consultant Oral and Maxillofacial Surgeon
University Hospitals Birmingham, UK

Prav Praveen FRCS, FDSRCS, FFDRCSI
Consultant Oral and Maxillofacial Surgeon
University Hospitals Birmingham, UK

Simon Van-Eeden FRCS Edin, FFDRCS Ireland, FRCS (OMFS)
Consultant Cleft Surgeon
Alderhey in the Park Children's Hospital, Liverpool, UK

About the examination

Components of Part 2 examination

The FRCS (Oral & Maxfacillofacial Surgery) Part 2 examination is a 2-day assessment. There is one day of examination interviews (the vivas), and one day of mock clinical consultations with patients. This book will help you prepare for the clinical component.

Potential scenarios

The patients brought in will be those treated by the team at the unit you are taking the examination at, so try to find out what types of patients they treat. It is unlikely, although not impossible, that some patients will be children.

Dress code and demeanour

You are advised to dress as if you would when performing a clinic, and in our experience candidates should dress as they would for the subsequent viva (i.e. a suit for men and the equivalent for woman).

Before you start the mock consultations, remove your jacket, roll up your sleeves and tuck in your tie. Remember to appear calm and confident; the examiners are deciding whether you would make an appropriate consultant colleague and addition to the specialty, so you must act the part.

Mark sheets

The current mark sheet can be downloaded from the Joint Committee of Intercollegiate Examinations website but this is subject to change. A grade of 6 is required to pass each station, and higher scores in some stations can compensate for lower scores in other stations. There is no 'immediate fail'.

Abbreviations

AAO-HNS	American Academy of Otolaryngology–Head and Neck Surgery
AAOMS	American Association of Oral and Maxillofacial Surgeons
ABCDE	Airway, Breathing, Circulation, Disability, Exposure
ACTH	Adrenocorticotropic hormone
AHI	Apnoea–Hypoapnoea Index
AJCC	American Joint Committee on Cancer
ALT	Anterolateral thigh
ANS	Anterior nasal spine
AOB	Anterior open bite
ASA	American Society of Anaesthesiologists
ATLS	Advanced Trauma Life Support
AVM	Arteriovenous malformation
BATS	British Association of TMJ Surgeons
BDD	Body dysmorphic disorder
BSSO	Bilateral sagittal split osteotomy
CBCT	Cone-beam computed tomography
CCG	Costochondral graft
CFNG	Cross-facial nerve grafts
CH	Condylar hyperplasia
CPAP	Continuous positive airway pressure
CSA	Circumflex scapular artery
CSF	Cerebrospinal fluid
CT	Computed tomography
CTA	Computed tomography angiography
CTLA-4	Cytotoxic T lymphocyte antigen-4
CTX	C-terminal cross-linking telopeptide
CUP	Cancer of unknown primary
DAHANCA	Danish Head and Neck Cancer
DCIA	Deep circumflex iliac artery
DCP	Dynamic compression plate
DE-ESCALATE	Determination of Epidermal growth factor receptor-inhibitor (cetuximab) versus Standard Chemotherapy (cisplatin) early And Late Toxicity Events
DFS	Disease-free survival
DICOM	Digital Imaging and Communications in Medicine
DMARDs	Disease-modifying antirheumatic drugs
DO	Distraction osteogenesis
DORs	Diagnostic odds ratios
DP	Deltopectoral
DSS	Disease-specific survival
EBRT	External beam radiotherapy

EBV	Epstein–Barr virus
ECS	Extracapsular spread
ECT	Electrochemotherapy
ED	Emergency department
END	Elective neck dissection
ESS	Epworth Sleepiness scale
ETV	Endoscopic third ventriculostomy
EUA	Examination under anaesthesia
FAMM	Facial artery myomucosal
FFP	Flaccid facial palsy
FMP	Frankfort Mandibular Plane
FMPA	Frankfort-mandibular plane angle
FNA	Fine-needle aspiration
FNAC	Fine-needle aspiration cytology
FNE	Fiberoptic nasoendoscopy
FOM	Floor of Mouth
FZ	Frontozygomatic
GA	General anaesthesia
GIT	Gastrointestinal tract
GSW	Gunshot wound
HA	Hyaluronic acid
HBO	Hyperbaric oxygen
HE	Hemimandibular elongation
HFM	Hemifacial microsomia
HH	Hemimandibular hyperplasia
HOPON	Hyperbaric oxygen for the prevention of osteoradionecrosis
HPV	Human papilloma virus
HRQoL	Health-related quality of life
IA	Inferior alveolar
IAN	Inferior alveolar nerve
IASI	Intra-articular steroid injection
ICP	Intracranial pressure
IMA	Internal mammary artery
IMAP	Internal mammary artery perforator
IMECC	Inframammary extended circumflex scapular
IMF	Intermaxillary Fixation
IMRT	Intensity-modulated radiotherapy
ISSVA	International Society for the Study of Vascular Anomalies
ITCs	Isolated tumour cells
LA	Local anaesthesia
LAFH	Lower anterior facial height
LIHNCS	Lugol's iodine in head and neck cancer surgery
LLC	Lower lateral cartilage

LP	Lichen planus
MACH-NC	Meta-analysis of chemotherapy in head and neck cancer
MACS	Minimal access cranial suspension
MALT	Mucosa-associated lymphoid tissue
MALToma	Mucosa-associated lymphoid tissue lymphoma
MCT	Medium-chain triglyceride
MDT	Multidisciplinary team
MLD	Margin limbal distance
MMF	Maxillary–mandibular fixation
MMO	Maximum mouth opening
MMPA	Maxillary–mandibular plane angle
MR	Magnetic resonance
MRA	Magnetic resonance angiography
MRONJ	Medication-related osteonecrosis of the jaw
MSAP	Medial sural artery perforator
MSLT	Multicenter Selective Lymphadenectomy Trial
mTOR	Mammalian target of rapamycin
NICE	National Institute for Health and Care Excellence
NOE	Naso-orbital-ethmoidal
NSAID	Nonsteroidal anti-inflammatory drug
OA	Osteoarthritis
OLP	Oral lichen planus
OPG	Orthopantomogram
OPSCC	Oropharyngeal squamous cell carcinoma
ORIF	Open reduction and internal fixation
ORN	Osteoradionecrosis
OS	Overall survival
OSA	Obstructive sleep apnoea
PA	Posteroanterior
PCI	Patient concerns inventory
PD-1	Programmed cell death 1
PDS	Personal data sheet
PEEK	Polyether ether ketone
PENTOCLO	Pentoxifylline, tocopherol and clodronate
PMMA	Polymethylmethacrylate
PMMC	Pectoralis major myocutaneous
PMR	Polymyalgia rheumatic
PNS	Posterior nasal spine
PTH	Parathyroid hormone
QoL	Quality of life
RCM	Reflectance confocal microscopy
RCT	Randomised Controlled Trial

RTOG/EORTC	Radiation Therapy Oncology Group and European Organisation for Research and Treatment of Cancer
SCC	Squamous cell carcinoma
SMAS	Superficial musculoaponeurotic system
SN	Sella to nasion
SND	Selective neck dissection
SNLB	Sentinel lymph node biopsy
SORG	Strasbourg Osteosynthesis Research Group
SPECT	Single photon emission computed tomography
STIR	Short tau inversion recovery
SSMDT	Specialist skin cancer multidisciplinary teams
STS	Sodium tetradecyl sulphate
TAFH	Total anterior face height
TDAA	Thoracodorsal angular artery
TJR	Total joint replacement
TLM	Transoral laser microsurgery
TMD	Temporomandibular disorders
TMI	Total mucosal irradiation
TMJ	Temperomandibular joint
TND	Therapeutic neck dissection
TORS	Transoral robotic surgery
TPF	Temporalis/temporoparietal fascia
ULC	Upper lateral cartilage
US	Ultrasonography
VPI	Velopharyngeal insufficiency
VSS	Vertical subsigmoid osteotomy
ZF	Zygomaticofrontal
ZMC	Zygomaticomaxillary complex

Acknowledgements

I would like to thank my loving family for the support that they have given me when military and clinical commitments have kept me away from them. I remain indebted to those who have mentored and guided me over the years, in particular Andrew Gibbons, Rhodri Williams, Andrew Monaghan and David Powers.

Johno Breeze

I would like to express my gratitude to all the trainers who believed in me and inspired me throughout my basic and higher surgical training, in particular the Training Programme Director for the West Midlands, Rhodri Williams, who was kind enough to join us as senior supervising editor in this endeavour. I would like to thank my section co-authors Satyesh Parmar, Jason Green and Demetrius Evriviades, who have patiently reviewed and commented on countless rough drafts. I would also like to thank the following trainers on the TIG Fellowships – Mark Henley, Jonathan Pollock, Lorraine Abercrombie, Howard Peach, Donald Dewar, Daniel Wilks and Jenny Goodenough – who were kind enough to "adopt" me as one of the first Maxillofacial trainees to undertake these periods of advanced training. My special thanks also to Alan Attard and Bernie Speculand, who along with Jason Green inspired a love of TMJ surgery in me, and a realisation of the life-changing effects it can achieve. Finally, but perhaps most importantly, I would like to acknowledge the support and love of my wife Roxy and our two beautiful children, Miles and Sienna. Without them, none of it would be worthwhile.

Ross Elledge

I would like to thank both Johno Breeze and Ross Elledge for asking me to be the senior editor for this book and who have worked tirelessly on it. Without their energy this project would not have been completed. I would also like to thank all of the other authors who have been kind enough to give up their time to help write and illustrate each and every chapter. I do believe that this is a comprehensive overview of what is required by a trainee approaching their FRCS(OMFS) and it's a real reflection of the quality of the clinicians who have helped in its creation. I would also like to thank Steffan Clements and his colleagues at JP Medical who were willing to put their faith in the book and been patient during its making.

Rhodri Williams

Chapter 1

Dentoalveolar surgery

SHORT CASES

1. Coronectomy
2. Displaced tooth root and CBCT
3. Management of an unerupted canine
4. Third molar assessment
5. Lip numbness following implant placement
6. Post-traumatic alveolar ridge and bone grafts

LONG CASE

7. Tongue numbness following third molar extraction

Short case 1: Coronectomy

This patient presents with the OPG shown in the figure, having been referred by their dentist for left-sided toothache.

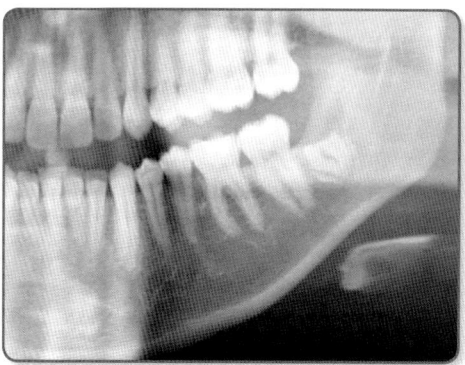

1.1 Question
What are the key points in the history?

Answer
- Pain: sharp/dull, exacerbating factors, duration
- Time after surgery for mandibular third molar
- Planned coronectomy (Box A) or intraoperative decision
- Medical health and drug history
- Social history: occupation and hobbies

1.2 Question
It is 3 weeks since they had surgery to their lower third molar. What are the key points in the examination?

Answer
- Extraoral: swelling, mouth opening, altered sensation to lip
- Intraoral: surgical site healing, damage or pathology to adjacent teeth, altered sensation to tongue

1.3 Question
What can you gauge from this OPG?

Answer
- Decoronated left mandibular third molar
- Likely elective coronectomy (horizontally sectioned, even cut)
- No crown tissue and roots appear approximately 3 mm below alveolar crest
- Root tips in close proximity to IA nerve
- No obvious pathology to third molar or adjacent teeth

1.4 Question

What are the indications for coronectomy?

Answer

- High-risk tooth: close proximity between tooth and IA canal (Box B)
- High-risk patient: e.g. professional wind instrument player

1.5 Question

When is it not appropriate to perform a coronectomy?

Answer

- Infection involving roots of teeth (Box C)
- Caries involving tooth
- Deep horizontal impaction where sectioning crown endangers nerve
- Cannot remove all the enamel of tooth
- Planned orthodontics involving second molar teeth

1.6 Question

Would you use lingual nerve retraction?

Answer

- No evidence for or against lingual nerve retraction in coronectomy
- Most rational decision would be for same approach as for third molars
- No evidence that lingual nerve injury incidence different to extraction

1.7 Question

The patient is complaining of hot and cold sensitivity with an intermittent dull ache and wants the roots extracted. What is the cause and how would you manage it?

Answer

- Likely to be due to sensitivity from adjacent second molar if mucosal coverage over the coronectomy site
- Too early to recommend further surgery unless infection cannot be managed with antibiotics

1.8 Question

How would you approach patient follow-up?

Answer

- No official guidelines or agreed recommendations currently exist
- Unless symptomatic follow-up in 1 year with repeat imaging as most tooth movement occurs in the first year

> **Box A: Key surgical steps in coronectomy**
>
> - Tooth sectioned at 45° buccolingual direction
> - Crown reduced to 3 mm below crestal surface ensuring removal of all enamel tissue
> - Teeth/roots that become mobile during the procedure should be extracted
> - Suture to produce primary closure
> - Use of lingual retraction not agreed upon
> - Concurrent guided bony regeneration has low morbidity and may reduce root migration

> **Box B: The case for coronectomy based on randomised controlled trials**
>
> - Renton 2005: extraction (n = 102) versus coronectomy (n = 94). Nineteen percent temporary and 2% permanent IA nerve injuries in extraction group, none in coronectomy group
> - Leung 2009: extraction (n = 178) versus coronectomy (n = 171). Five percent temporary and 2% permanent nerve injury in extractions, 1% temporary and no permanent in coronectomies

> **Box C: The case against coronectomy**
>
> - The roots may become infected or migrate unfavourably
> - A radicular cyst may develop necessitating further surgery

Further reading

Leung YY, Cheung LK. Safety of coronectomy versus excision of wisdom teeth: a randomized controlled trial. Oral Surg Oral Med Oral Pathol Oral Radiol Endod 2009; 108:821–827.

Leung YY. Coronectomy of lower third molars with and without guided bony regeneration: a pilot study. Br J Oral Maxillofac Surg 2016; 54:155–159.

Renton T, Hankins M, Sproate C, et al. A randomised controlled clinical trial to compare the incidence of injury to the inferior alveolar nerve as a result of coronectomy and removal of mandibular third molars. Br J Oral Maxillofac Surg 2005; 43:7–12.

Short case 2: Displaced tooth root and CBCT

The patient shown in the figure has been referred by their dentist who is concerned that a root was displaced into the maxillary sinus during extraction a month ago.

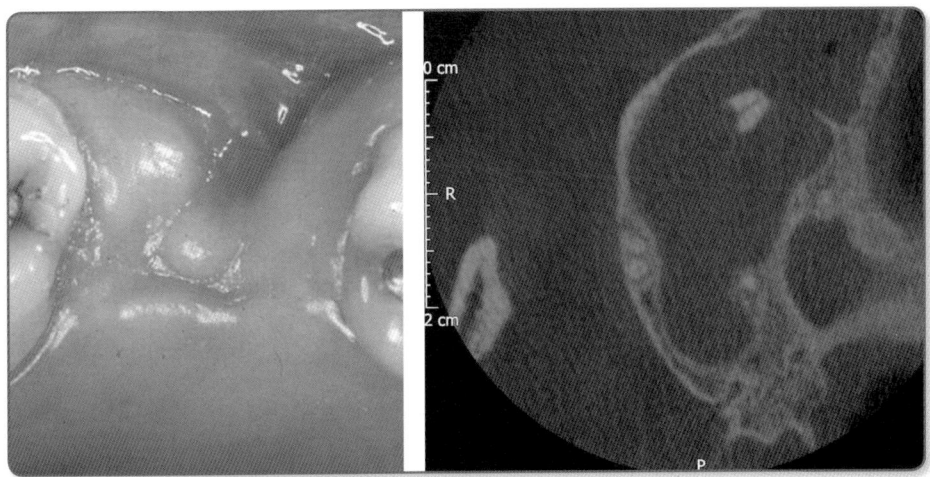

2.1 Question

What are the specific points from the patient's history?

Answer

- Which tooth surgically extracted and symptomatic preoperatively
- Nasal discharge or regurgitation/fluid reflux
- Bad taste in the mouth
- Bad smell
- Cheek pain or swelling
- Pain from other teeth
- Medical and drug history
- Social history: smoking

2.2 Question

What are the key points to ascertain in the examination?

Answer

- Extraoral: cheek swelling and erythema, altered sensation
- Intraoral: extraction site healing, infection, communication, discharge, bubbling

2.3 Question

The OPG demonstrates no obvious retained root. How would you manage an asymptomatic patient?

Answer

- An asymptomatic patient can be discharged, and reviewed again if they become symptomatic

2.4 Question

Would you request a CBCT?

Answer

- In the absence of clinical symptoms most clinicians would not request an additional CBCT as unlikely to change management and has radiation dose and reporting implications (Boxes B-D)
- In absence of clinical symptoms most clinicians would not request an additional CBCT as unlikely to change management
- CBCT indicated potentially instead of OPG in first place

2.5 Question

The patient is referred back by the dentist with this scan as the patient wants an implant. What do you see?

Answer

- Axial CBCT slice
- A retained root in the right maxillary sinus

2.6 Question

What are the options for a retained root in the maxillary sinus?

Answer

- Conservative: if asymptomatic
- Surgical removal using Caldwell-Luc approach
- Endoscopic retrieval via nose into sinus

2.7 Question

The patient's dentist won't place an implant until the root is removed from the sinus. What would you do?

Answer

- If patient asymptomatic no contraindication to implant placement and leaving root in situ
- If patient symptomatic or sinus lift required, then root removal via Caldwell-Luc approach recommended

Box A: Determinants of dose in CBCT

- Field of view size
- Image resolution
- Age of device
- Scanning protocol

Box B: Rule of thumb comparisons using modern imaging equipment (post 2015)

- Single periapical: 4 µSv
- Lateral cephalogram: 6 µSv
- OPG: 12 µSv
- Low-resolution CBCT single tooth: 18 µSv
- High-resolution CBCT maxilla + mandible: 200 µSv
- 32 row/64-slice MultiDetector CT single jaw: 360 µSv
- Daily background radiation dose in UK: 3 µSv

Box C: Situations when a CBCT is not suitable for dentoalveolar assessment

- When plain films alone will suffice: doses should be as low as reasonably achievable (ALARA)
- When a standard CT is required, e.g. to assess soft tissue

Box D: Clinicians who can request and report a CBCT scan

- Prescribers are mandated by the Health and Safety Executive to have undertaken Core Training in CBCT
- Reporters are recommended (but not yet mandated) to have additional training if scans incorporate the base of skull, temporal bones, neck and spine regions

Further reading

Brown J, Jacobs R, Levring Jäghagen E, et al. Basic training requirements for the use of dental CBCT by dentists: a position paper prepared by the European Academy of DentoMaxilloFacial Radiology. Dentomaxillofac Radiol 2014; 43:20130291.

Health and Safety Executive. Ionising Radiation (Medical Exposure) Regulations 2017. Health Protection Agency. Guidance on the safe use of cone beam CT equipment. London: Health Protection Agency, 2010.

Short case 3: Management of an unerupted canine

The patient shown in the figure has been referred by your orthodontist for exposure and bonding of the upper left canine.

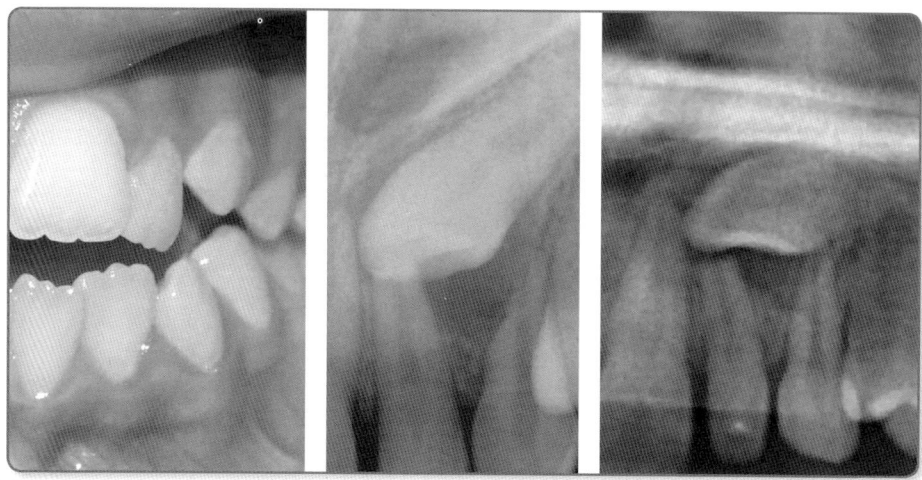

3.1 Question
What are the key points in the history?

Answer

- Age
- Previous and planned extractions
- Medical contraindications to surgery
- Patient's request: exposure, extraction, prolonged orthodontics

3.2 Question
What are the key points in the examination?

Answer

- Skeletal and dental discrepancy: to determine if orthognathic treatment or orthodontic camouflage best
- Palpable unerupted canine
- Lateral incisor proclination (canine likely buccal) or retroclination (canine likely palatal)
- Mobility of upper lateral and deciduous canine: prognosis of these teeth
- Crowding: may necessitate extractions
- Caries risk and periodontal health: contraindications to treatment

Short case 3 Management of an unerupted canine

3.3 **Question 3.4**

The orthodontist has sent in these radiographs (Box A). What technique is this and where is the canine?

Answer

- Two periapical films used for horizontal parallax (Box B)
- Position inferred using Same Lingual Opposite Buccal (SLOB) acronym
- Tooth has not moved between radiographs suggesting it is in line with arch

3.4 **Question**

Would you request an additional CBCT and if so why?

Answer

- Yes, there is evidence of root resorption (Box C)
- CBCT most use when tooth does not move on parallax
- Means it is closest to arch and therefore tooth roots

3.5 **Question**

If the patient did not have up-to-date imaging, would you have gone straight for CBCT?

Answer

- Periapical in conjunction with OPG suitable for vast majority of canine assessment
- Low resolution CBCT with strictly field of view taken on modern device has a dose only twice that of periapical plus OPG (approximately 20 μSv versus 40 μSv)

3.6 **Question**

Do you agree that expose and bonding is the best scenario?

Answer

- The canine is not in a favourable position according to McSherry (Box D)
- Both permanent lateral incisor and deciduous canine have poor long-term prognosis
- Patient will lose little from attempt at expose and bonding

3.7 **Question**

What potential risks of surgery would you advise the patient to expect?

Answer

- Damage to the adjacent teeth
- Exposed canine does not move (ankylosis)
- Debonding of bracket/chain
- Further treatment

> **Box A: The role of radiology in canine orthodontic assessment**
> - To identify the position of the canine to determine if amenable to expose and bond
> - Identify position of canine to determine surgical approach
> - To determine pathology with tooth (e.g. cyst) or adjacent teeth (e.g. resorption)

> **Box B: Combinations of imaging in canine parallax**
> - Two periapicals (horizontal parallax)
> - An OPG (10° to the horizontal) and a periapical (vertical parallax)
> - An OPG and upper occlusal (vertical parallax)
> - Cone Beam CT

> **Box C: Indications for additional CBCT in canine orthodontic assessment**
> - Assessment of ankylosis prior to expose and bonding
> - Assessment of existing damage of teeth adjacent to the canine
> - Unsure of position of canine
> - Assessment of canine morphology

> **Box D: Predictions for likelihood of assisted eruption (McSherry)**
> - Overlap of incisor: increased overlap has a poor prognosis
> - Angulation of tooth: horizontal angulation has a poor prognosis
> - Vertical height crown: the higher up the canine the worse the prognosis
> - Position of the canine root apex: a laterally positioned apex has a poor prognosis

Further reading

Husain J, Burden D, McSherry P, Morris D, Allen M. National clinical guidelines for management of the palatally ectopic maxillary canine. Br Dent J 2012; 213:171–176.

McSherry PF. The ectopic maxillary canine: a review. Br J Orthodo 1998; 25:209–216.

Parkin N, Benson PE, Thind B, et al. Open versus closed surgical exposure of canine teeth that are displaced in the roof of the mouth. Cochrane Database Syst Rev 2017; 8:CD006966.

Short case 4: Third molar assessment

The patient shown in the figure has been referred by the dentist for pain in the left lower third molar.

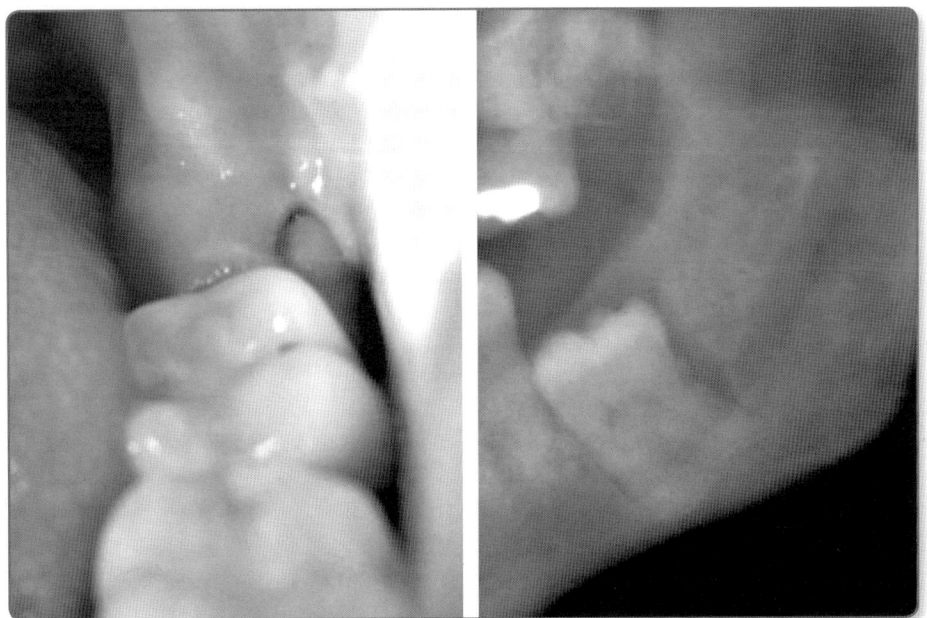

4.1 Question

What are the key points from the patient's history?

Answer

- Symptoms tailored from the National Institute of Clinical Excellence (NICE) guidelines for extraction (Box A)
- Fitness for surgery
- Drug history

4.2 Question

They have had multiple episodes of pericoronitis. How will you examine the patient?

Answer

- Degree of eruption of third molar
- Inflammation of operculum
- Caries in second molar tooth
- Upper third molar impinging on operculum
- Restorations present in neighbouring teeth (risk of damage during extraction)

4.3 Question

What comments do you have on the OPG (right image) taken at the appointment?

Answer

- Deep vertical impaction of third molar
- Radiolucent band suggesting close proximity to inferior alveolar nerve (Box B)
- No obvious pathology in third or second molar
- Curved mesial root

4.4 Question

Is there anything else you would undertake in the assessment to alter your management?

Answer

- Request a CBCT scan (Box C)
- Determine the exact relation of the nerve to the tooth
- Guide the position of surgical cuts

4.5 Question

CBCT shows the nerve to be separate and buccal to the tooth. What is your proposed treatment and why?

Answer

- Surgical extraction
- Coronectomy requires sectioning crown from buccal aspect near nerve

4.6 Question

The patient agrees to surgical extraction. What potential risks would you advise the patient to expect?

Answer

- Higher risk of damage to inferior alveolar and lingual nerves than conventional extraction for less deeply impacted tooth (Box D)
- Pathological fracture necessitating intraoperative fixation

4.7 Question

What are the options for extraction?

Answer

- Conventional intra approach without using lingual split technique
- Lingual split good for lingually-placed tooth but still requires buccal bone removal with chisel where nerve is situated
- Consider sagittal split osteotomy if very deeply positioned
- In rare cases extraoral approach used; leaves scar and risks marginal mandibular nerve but may be easier to access tooth if very displaced, e.g. ascending mandibular ramus

4.8 Question

How would you undertake the extraction?

Answer

- Raise buccal and lingual flaps
- Remove distal and mesial bone with bur
- Section tooth vertically from lingual to buccal with bur, but stop 2/3 way through
- Complete sectioning of tooth with an osteotome or elevator

Box A: The NICE guidelines for extraction of third molars comprise

- Unrestorable caries in third molar (but not the second)
- Periapical pathology (e.g. cyst)
- Tooth fracture
- Two mild episodes of pericoronitis or one severe
- Osteomyelitis
- Orthognathic surgery
- Oncological resection

Box B: Signs of close proximity on OPG in order of risk.

- Radiolucent band across root (highest risk)
- Deviation of canal
- Narrowing of canal
- Loss of the canal tramlines

Box C: Indications for CBCT in third molar assessment

- Both upper and lower cortices of the IAN canal being overlapped by the tooth root
- Signs of close proximity on the OPG

Box D: Incidences for nerve injury following third molar extraction

- Inferior alveolar: temporary (20%) and permanent (1%)
- Lingual: temporary (10%) and permanent (0.5%)

Further reading

Catherine Z, Scolozzi P. Mandibular Sagittal Split Osteotomy for Removal of Impacted Mandibular Teeth: Indications, Surgical Pitfalls, and Final Outcome. J Oral Maxillofac Surg 2017; 75:915–923.

Cheung LK, Leung YY, Chow LK, et al. Incidence of neurosensory deficits and recovery after lower third molar surgery: a prospective clinical study of 4338 cases. Int J Oral Maxillofac Surg 2010; 39:320–326.

National Institute for Health and Clinical Excellence. Guidance on the Extraction of Wisdom Teeth. Technology appraisal guidance TA1. London: NICE, 2000.

Short case 5: Lip numbness following implant placement

This patient shown in the figure has been sent to you by their dentist with problems following implants.

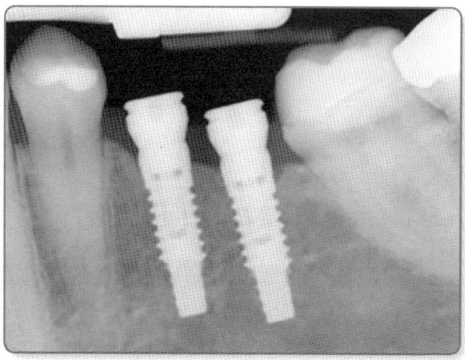

5.1 Question

What are the key points in the history?

Answer

- First or second stage of implants
- Time since placement
- Complications: biological and technical (Box A)
- Medical history including contraindications to implant placement (Box B)
- Drug and social history

5.2 Question

First-stage implants were placed 1 week ago by a different clinician to their usual dentist. How you would examine the patient?

Answer

- Extraoral: general health, swelling, mouth opening
- Intraoral: closure of mucosa
- Generic implant assessment (Box C)

5.3 Question

The patient was provided with this radiograph by their dentist prior to planned restoration. What can you see?

Answer

- A periapical radiograph showing two implants in left premolar region
- Implants appear transmucosal
- Implants are too close together (Box D)
- Relationship to nerve canal not clear

5.4 Question

What would be the next step in management?

Answer

- Request an OPG (or CBCT) to better demonstrate relationship of implant to canal

5.5 Question

The OPG demonstrates the canal appears to be well away from the implants. How would you advise the patient?

Answer

- Nerve may have been damaged during implant preparation
- Implant placement should be >2 mm above the canal
- Anterior loop may be up to 5 mm in front of the mental foramen
- Recommend patient has discussion with clinician who placed implants

5.6 Question

The patient does not want to see the clinician who placed the implants. How would you manage the patient going forward and why?

Answer

- Request a CBCT to relate canal position to the implant
- A CBCT may show bone loss from implant preparation

5.7 Question

The CBCT shows the implant is >2 mm lateral to the canal. How would you manage the patient?

Answer

If <36 hours after implant placement, evidence supports removal of both implants in conjunction with oral steroids and nonsteroidal anti-inflammatory drug

5.8 Question

If it was 1 week after placement, what would you tell the patient about the long-term prognosis?

Answer

- No evidence to support removal of implant or adjunctive medications
- Resolution of any numbness unpredictable
- Five-year survival of each implant >95% (Box E)

Box A: Potential complications of implant placement

Biological
- Mucositis: reversible peri-implant inflammation
- Peri-implantitis: nonreversible with bone loss
- Periimplant abscess
- Lip and chin numbness

Technical
- Fractures: fixture, screw, abutment, veneer, metal framework
- Loosening: screw, abutment
- Loss of retention: fracture of luting cement

Box B: Contraindications to implant placement

Absolute
- Recent cardiac valve replacement
- Untreated dental disease
- Mucosal disease (e.g. erosive LP)
- Active cancer therapy
- Intravenous bisphosphonates: poor evidence to support this

Relative
- Smoking: risk is doubled
- Oral bisphosphonates: risk normalises after 3 years
- Previous radiotherapy
- Immunosuppression
- Diabetes: risk normalises with good glycemic control
- Bone disorders: osteoporosis (reduces primary stability)
- Bruxism: due to micromovement

Box C: Generic implant examination

Extraoral
- Implant visibility at rest and smiling
- Mouth opening
- Temporomandibular joint

Intraoral
- Occlusion
- Teeth present
- Ridge form where implant being placed (Cawood and Howell)
- Caries risk assessment
- Periodontal health
- Gingival biotype

> **Box D: Minimum distances between implants and adjacent teeth**
> - Mesiodistal: 1.5 mm from adjacent tooth, 3 mm from adjacent implant
> - Buccolingual: implant should be 3 mm smaller (i.e. 1.5 mm on buccal and lingual sides)
> - Apicocoronal: 2 mm above canal or maxillary sinus
> - Interarch: >7 mm

> **Box E: Five-year survival of a single implant in the mandible**
> - No risk factors: >98%
> - Placed after radiation: 97%
> - Before radiation: 95%

Further reading

Khawaja N, Renton T. Case studies on implant removal influencing the resolution of inferior alveolar nerve injury. Br Dent J 2009; 206:365–370.

Short case 6: Post-traumatic alveolar ridge and bone grafts

The patient shown in the figure has been struggling to eat since an injury 2 years ago.

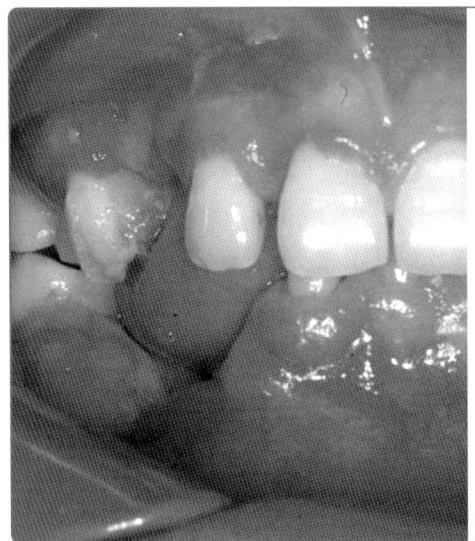
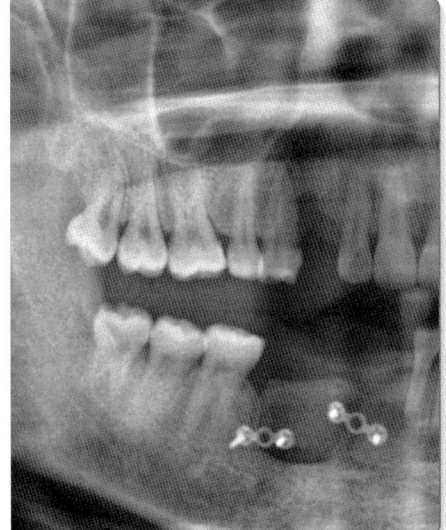

6.1 Question

How would you examine them?

Answer

Extraoral
- Cutaneous involvement including sinus tract

Intraoral
- Oral hygiene
- Ridge shape and form
- Prognosis of adjacent teeth
- Occlusion

6.2 Question

Is there a classification that would help describe the defect to the alveolar ridge?

Answer
- Nontraumatic defects are best described using the Cawood and Howell classification (Box A)
- This case demonstrates loss of horizontal and vertical bone
- No obvious loss of sulcus depth

6.3 Question

How would you assess the patient further and why?

Answer

- OPG and periapical radiographs: assess prognosis of adjacent teeth
- CT scan: height of residual bone, continuity of bone, retained metalwork or foreign bodies
- Medical history, smoking history

6.4 Question

What are the treatment options for this patient?

Answer

- Removable prosthesis
- Fixed bridge: long span
- Implant retained removable or fixed prosthesis: needs bone augmentation
- Short implants: increasing evidence for 7 mm and even 4 mm length in posterior mandible

6.5 Question

What are the options for augmentation?

Answer

- Nonvascularised autogenous bone graft (Box B): onlay or ridge split
- Vascularised bone graft
- Distraction
- Allograft/xenograft/alloplast plus titanium mesh/resorbable membrane/bone morphogenic protein

6.6 Question

What can you infer from the given radiograph?

Answer

- OPG showing a corticocancellous block graft
- Graft secured with miniplates
- Graft likely to be nonvascularised

6.7 Question

How does a corticocancellous graft form new bone compared to bone substitutes?

Answer

- Autogenous bone: osteogenesis, osteoinduction and osteoconduction (Box C)
- Allograft/xenograft: osteoinductive and osteoconductive capabilities
- Alloplastic: osteoconductive

6.8 Question

What are the problems with performing a block graft?

Answer
- Achieving mucosal coverage of graft: graft may fail
- Loss of sulcal depth: may require vestibuloplasty

Box A: Classification of alveolar ridge defects (Cawood and Howell)

- Class 1: dentate (normal ridge)
- Class II: postextraction
- Class III: adequate height and width
- Class IV: adequate height, inadequate width (knife-edge ridge)
- Class V: inadequate height, inadequate width (flat ridge)
- Class VI: loss of alveolar and basal bone (submerged ridge)

Box B: Materials used for guided bone regeneration

- Autogenous bone: mandibular ramus, mandibular symphysis, maxillary tuberosity, iliac crest, calvarium, rib, tibia
- Allografts: freeze dried demineralised bone
- Alloplastic: hydroxyapatite, and tricalcium phosphate

Box C: Methods of new bone formation

- Osteoconduction: scaffold for new bone from adjacent living bone
- Osteoinduction: mediators that stimulate recipient site cells to differentiate into osteoblasts, e.g. bone morphogenic proteins
- Osteogenesis: vital osteoblasts originating from the bone graft material produce bone

Further reading

Bolle C, Felice P, Barausse C, et al. 4 mm long vs longer implants in augmented bone in posterior atrophic jaws: 1-year post-loading results from a multicentre randomised controlled trial. Eur J Oral Implantol 2018; 11:31–47.

Cawood J, Howell R. A classification of the edentulous jaws. Int J Oral Maxillofac Surg 1988; 17:232–236.

Hart KL, Bowles D. Reconstruction of alveolar defects using titanium-reinforced porous polyethylene as a containment device for recombinant human bone morphogenetic protein. J Oral Maxillofac Surg 2012; 70:811–820.

Long case 7: Tongue numbness following third molar extraction

The patient shown in the figure had a tooth extracted 4 weeks ago and returns with numbness.

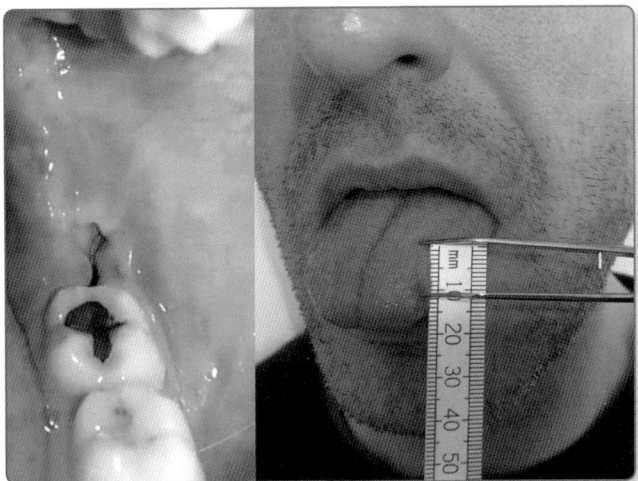

7.1 Scenario
Assess them and provide your proposed management plan (Box A).

7.2 Preparation
- Use the time to introduce yourself, clean your hands and obtain consent to assess.
- Position the patient and try to come to a spot diagnosis

7.3 History
- Altered sensation: hypoesthesia, anaesthesia, analgesia, dysaesthesia, paraesthesia (Box B)
- Altered taste
- Level of improvement
- Effect on speech, eating and quality of life

7.4 Examination
- Wound site: erythema, pus or pain on palpation
- Light touch: von Frey hair
- Two-point discrimination: dental tweezers
- State that you would ideally assess pain and taste
- Note that the Medical Research Council grading system is not useful in clinical practice

7.5 Investigations

- Preoperative OPG: assess difficulty of original extraction
- Read operation notes for technique used and difficulty
- Postoperative CBCT: to assess bone defect lingually from drilling or surgery
- Photographs: with area of sensation loss marked out
- Nerve conduction studies

7.6 Management plan

- Thank the patient and summarise your findings
- Postulate where the nerve may potentially have been damaged (Box C)
- Suitability for surgery
- Discuss with examiner recommended surgery (Box D)
- Treatment options for a late presentation
- Arguments for and against lingual retraction (Box E)

Box A: Concept of a dentoalveolar long case

- A 15-minute assessment likely encompassing the structure above
- It would inevitably include another component such as treatment complications (fracture, numbness), an unsuspected pathology, or spreading dentofacial infection

---

Box B: Commonly used descriptions of sensation

- Anaesthesia: absence of touch appreciation
- Hypoesthesia: reduced touch appreciation
- Analgesia: absence of pain appreciation
- Paraesthesia: abnormal sensations perceived without specific stimulation
- Dysaesthesia: painful sensation (often burning) elicited by a nonpainful stimulus

---

Box C: Where might the nerve have been damaged?

- Directly from the needle during injection
- Local anaesthetic toxicity: 4% articaine has been described as causing a higher incidence of altered sensation following inferior alveolar blocks than 2% lidocaine
- Retraction during the raising of a lingual flap
- Stretching of the nerve due to lingual displacement of bone or tooth during extraction
- Direct damage from rotary cutting instrument or similar

Box D: Suggested management of lingual nerve injury

- Tension-free, primary repair of an injured nerve provides the most optimal result
- If this is not possible, autogenous nerve grafts can be used for acute injuries
- Delayed reconstruction of gaps of 3 cm or smaller can be performed with either autogenous nerve grafts or hollow conduits to bridge the defect

Box E: The argument for lingual retraction

- Retraction only required if removing bone lingually
- Incidences for lingual nerve injury in the literature are highly variable
- Higher rates of injury are likely to reflect experience of surgeon and poor placement of retractor
- Overall incidence of lingual nerve injury with retraction: temporary (10%) and permanent (0.5%)

Further reading

Dodson T, Kaban L. Recommendations for management of trigeminal nerve defects based on a critical appraisal of the literature. J Oral Maxillofac Surg 1997; 55:1380–1386.

Leung Y, Cheung L. Longitudinal Treatment Outcomes of Microsurgical Treatment of Neurosensory Deficit after Lower Third Molar Surgery: A Prospective Case Series. PLoS One 2016; 11:e0150149.

Robinson PP, Smith KG. A study on the efficacy of late lingual nerve repair. Br J Oral Maxillofac Surg 1996; 34:96–103.

Chapter 2

Head and neck oncological surgery

SHORT CASES

1. Oncology patient history
2. Examining the oncology patient
3. Computed tomography (CT) imaging
4. Magnetic resonance (MR) imaging
5. Ultrasound assessment of neck lumps
6. Unknown primary and PET scanning
7. Sentinel lymph node biopsy
8. Oropharyngeal cancer
9. Radial forearm flap
10. Fibula flap
11. Pectoralis major myocutaneous flap
12. Anterolateral thigh flap
13. Scapular flap
14. Neck dissection
15. Upper lip defect reconstruction
16. Radiotherapy

LONG CASE

17. Maxillectomy and DCIA flap

Short case 1: Oncology patient history

You are asked to assess a patient who has recently had surgery for oral cancer.

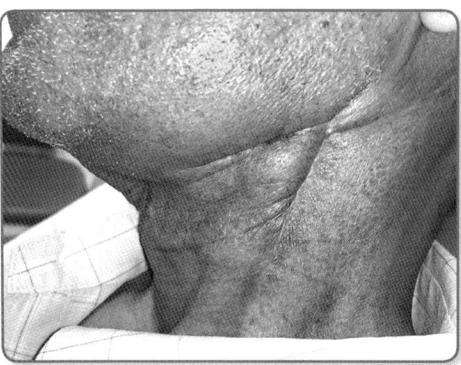

1.1 Question

How would you structure the history?

Answer

- Presenting complaint
- Previous treatment: surgical, radiotherapy, chemotherapy
- Complications of treatment
- Nature of surgery: incision type, reconstruction source
- Quality of life (QoL)
- Medical comorbidities
- Social history
- Focus on treatment to date, including nature of any ablative and reconstructive surgery and any adjuvant treatment received
- Explore comorbidities and their impact on the choice of treatment received and postoperative recovery

1.2 Question

What are the complications of treatment?

Answer

- Ask open questions such as "Have you had any ongoing issues as a result of your treatment?"
- Focus on particular areas of concern
- Speech and swallow
- Mouth opening
- Previous radiotherapy: dose and location (osteoradionecrosis)
- Prosthodontic rehabilitation

- Xerostomia
- Dietary intake and need for nutritional support

1.3 Question
What are the key points to explore in the patient's social history?

Answer
- Alcohol and smoking
- Cultural habits: betel nut, paan, chewing tobacco
- Human papillomavirus (HPV) status and other risk factors (Box A)
- Potentially malignant conditions, e.g. lichen planus
- Family support

1.4 Question
How would you ask about QoL?

Answer
- Health-related quality of life (HRQoL) as judged by a patient is equally as important as surgeon-reported outcomes
- Multiple validated QoL assessment tools exist (Box B)
- 20–30% of patients will experience a significant depressive episode at least once during their illness which may be missed at consultation (Box C)

Box A: Human papillomavirus

- HPV high-risk types are significantly associated with oropharyngeal squamous cell carcinoma (OPSCC)
- Transmission may be spread via oral sexual behavior and the number of lifetime sexual partners increases the risk for an HPV-positive head and neck cancer
- With better locoregional control and overall survival in HPV-OPSCC, current trials are exploring de-intensification of treatment (DE-ESCALATE) and a possible therapeutic role for the HPV vaccine (HARE-40)

Box B: Quality of life (QoL)

- There are over 75 QoL tools available in oncology, with generic scales (e.g. EuroQol, SF-36, etc) and specific ones (e.g. Fact-H&N) available
- Generic scales often explore areas such as mobility, self-care, daily activities, social interaction, psychosexual health
- Head and neck cancer specific ones examine areas such as appearance, mastication, speech, shoulder dysfunction, taste and saliva
- The University of Washington Questionnaire (UW-QoL) and QLQ-H&N35 are the most well cited scales used

> **Box C: The patient-guided consultation**
> - There is evidence to suggest that a combination of a rushed consultation in combination with possible low self-esteem in head and neck patients may mean that the most pertinent issues are not explored
> - Rogers et al. (2009) developed a Patient Concerns Inventory (PCI) to circumvent this and enable patients to tailor the consultation to meet their expectations
> - The commonest issues raised were fear of recurrence (37%), dental health (27%) and eating (24%)

Further reading

Heutte N, Plisson L, Lange M, et al. Quality of life tools in head and neck oncology. Eur Ann Otorhinolaryngol Head Neck Dis 2014; 131:33–47.

Kanatas A, Ghazali N, Lowe D, Rogers SN. The identification of mood and anxiety concerns using the patients concerns inventory following head and neck cancer. Int J Oral Maxillofac Surg 2012; 41:429–436.

Lassen P, Primdahl H, Johansen J, et al. Impact of HPV-associated p16-expression on radiotherapy outcome in advanced oropharynx and non-oropharynx cancer. Radiother Oncol 2014; 113:310–316.

Rogers SN, El-Sheikha J, Lowe D. The development of a Patients Concerns Inventory (PCI) to help reveal patient concerns in the head and neck clinic. Oral Oncol 2009; 45:555–561.

Short case 2: Examining the oncology patient

This patient with recently treated head and neck cancer has returned to clinic for a follow up

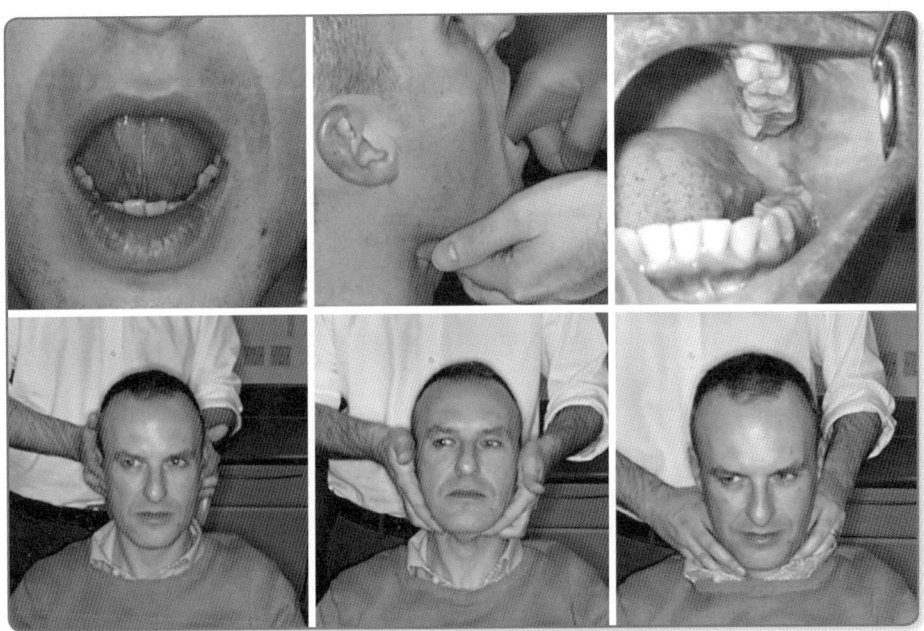

2.1 Question

How would you structure the examination as demonstrated in the figure?

Answer
- Positioning
- End of the bed
- Intraoral
- Extraoral
- Peripheral

2.2 Question

How would you position the patient?

Answer
- Sit patient in chair
- Remove, roll up or loosen any clothing required to examine neck and tissue donor sites
- Remove any prostheses (dentures, ocular)

2.3 Question

How would you conduct an intraoral examination?

Answer

- Examine oral cavity and oropharynx
- Determine resection location
- Determine reconstruction type: none, soft tissue, hard tissue, combination
- Skin paddles or mucosalised muscle-only flaps
- Classify any hard tissue defects
- Look for evidence of recurrence
- Osteoradionecrosis
- Consider adjuncts to assessment of margins (Box A)

2.4 Question

How would you conduct an extraoral examination?

Answer

- Palpate cervical lymph nodes: including occipital and level V
- Palpate parotid glands from behind patient
- Inspect: scar types neck dissection approach design (Box B), lip split mandibulotomy (Box C), tracheostomy
- Facial weakness (e.g. marginal mandibular weakness)
- Shoulder weakness/stiffness
- Skin numbness: lip, earlobe (greater auricular nerve)
- Stigmata of radiotherapy

2.5 Question

How would you perform a peripheral examination?

Answer

- Inspect soft tissue donor sites: radial, ALT
- Inspect hard tissue donor sites: scapula, fibula, iliac crest
- Ask patient to mobilise hard tissue donor sites, e.g. walking postfibula

2.6 Question

Are there any other assessments you would want to do?

Answer

- Speech: dysphagia/dysarthria from tethering of the tongue, velopharyngeal incompetence in soft palate reconstructions or persistent oroantral fistula
- Swallowing: glass of water

2.7 Question

How would you complete the assessment?

Answer

- Perform flexible nasendoscopy (FNE) if appropriate to examine aerodigestive tract and larynx

- If cervical lymphadenopathy is felt request further investigations, e.g. ultrasound, fine needle aspirate cytology
- Beware ptotic and/or obstructed submandibular gland following floor of mouth resections in early-stage tumours.

Box A: Lugol's iodine and the limits of human capability in examination

- Clinical examination of the neck is reported to be 70% sensitive for lymphadenopathy.
- The same limitations apply for examination of the oral cavity
- In an effort to increase accuracy, toluidine blue, Lugol's iodine and whitening of the oral mucosa with acetic acid have all been employed to differentiate intraepithelial neoplasia/dysplasia from benign tissue
- This has been employed in guiding resection margins in oral cancer with a better negative margin rate seen in the LIHNCS trial as described by McCaul et al.
- The iKnife may be the next step in intraoperative margin identification as described by Dhanda et al.

Box B: Neck dissection scars

- You should be familiar with the following designs: MacFee, Crile's, Schobinger, hockey stick', 'apron', Conley/Schechter, Hayes Martin, triradiate

---

Box C: Transoral robotic surgery (TORS) versus the lip split mandibulotomy

- Access to oropharyngeal tumours often means a lip split mandibulotomy
- Potential complications including a visible scar, notching of the vermillion and the potential for plate failure, osteoradionecrosis and nonunion at the osteotomy site
- Transoral robotic surgery (TORS) with equipment such as the da Vinci Surgical System enables resection of oropharyngeal squamous cell carcinomas (OPSCCs) and microvascular free flap reconstruction
- When seeing a patient who has undergone a lip split mandibulotomy, the merits of TORS may be mentioned
- It particularly finds its place in early stage OPSCC where it provides comparable locoregional control to radiotherapy

Further reading

Balsundaram I, Al-Hadad I, Parmar S. Recent advances in reconstructive oral and maxillofacial surgery. Br J Oral Maxillofac Surg 2012; 50:695–705.

Dhanda J, et al. iKnife rapid evaporative ionization mass spectrometry (REIMS) technology in head and neck surgery. An ex vivo feasibility study. Br J Oral Maxillofac Surg 2017; 55:e61–85.

McCaul JA, Cymerman JA, Hislop S, et al. LIHNCS - Lugol's iodine in head and neck cancer surgery: a multicentre, randomised controlled trial assessing the effectiveness of Lugol's iodine to assist excision of moderate dysplasia, severe dysplasia and carcinoma in situ at mucosal resection margins of oral and oropharyngeal squamous cell carcinoma: study protocol for a randomised controlled trial. Trials 2013; 14:310.

Short case 3: Computed tomography (CT) imaging

This figure shows an example of a CT.

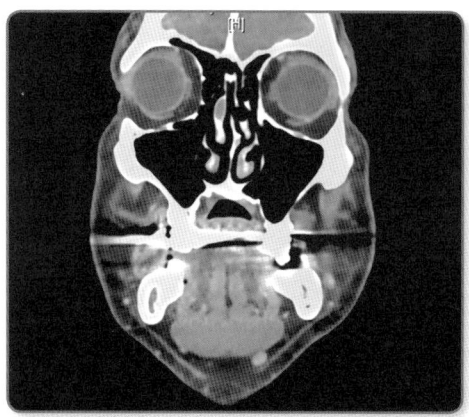

3.1 Question

How effective is CT in assessing lymphadenopathy?

Answer

- Provides limited soft tissue resolution but good bone detail (e.g. mandibular invasion, base of skull)
- Has sensitivity of 54–95% and specificity of 39–100% when looking for metastatic cervical lymphadenopathy

3.2 Question

What is the role of a CT of the thorax in staging?

Answer

- Frequency of coincident thoracic malignancy is reported as between 3.5% and 17% in patients with head and neck cancer
- Bisase et al. reported that when restricting this to patients with T1–T2 N0 tumours, only 3.8% (n = 2) had an 'abnormality' on chest CT
- In neither of the cases in this series did this have an impact on treatment decisions and both abnormalities were visible on plain film radiography
- Given the radiation dose of CT (Box A), they called for rationalising the routine use of CT in staging
- Latest UK guidelines recommend CT thorax in staging

3.3 Question

What is the role of CT in assessing bone involvement of the primary?

Answer

- Valuable in demonstrating subtle cortical erosions

- Findings indicative of possible bone invasion on CT include cortical erosion, aggressive periosteal reaction, abnormal attenuation in bone marrow and pathological fractures

3.4 Question

What are the advantages and disadvantages of CT compared with MRI?

Answer

- CT image quality affected by dental amalgam artifact – less impact on MRI
- CT significantly quicker to perform than MRI
- Speed of procedure is a key consideration for patients with upper aerodigestive tract tumours with difficulty lying flat for any length of time
- CT is less sensitive than MR for assessing bone marrow involvement

3.5 Question

How can you better examine buccal mucosa primaries on CT?

Answer

- Exhalation against resistance puffs the cheeks outwards to better demonstrate this area
- Clinical examination key in this area
- Radiological findings serve as an adjunct and more meaningfully determining nodal status and presence/absence of distant metastases

---

Box A: CT thorax radiation doses

- The radiation dose of a plain chest film (CXR) is 0.02 mSV
- A conventional CT may be over 8 mSV
- A spiral CT up to 12 mSV, effectively the equivalent of 600 chest films
- This translates to 20–50 mGy and a 13% increase in the risk of breast cancer

---

Further reading

Bisase B, Kerawala C, Lee J. The role of computed tomography of the chest in the staging of early squamous cell carcinoma of the tongue. Br J Oral Maxillofac Surg 2008; 46:367–369.

de Bondt RBJ, Nelemans PJ, Hofman PA, et al. Detection of lymph node metastases in head and neck cancer: a meta-analysis comparing US, USgFNAC, CT and MR imaging. Eur J Radiol 2007; 64:266–272.

Lewis-Jones H, Colley S, Gibson D. Imaging in head and neck cancer: United Kingdom National Multidisciplinary Guidelines. J Laryngol Otol 2016; 130:S28–S31.

Trotta BM, Pease CS, Rasamny JJ, et al. Oral cavity and oropharyngeal squamous cell cancer: key imaging findings for staging and treatment planning. Radiographics 2011; 31:339–354.

Short case 4: Magnetic resonance (MR) imaging

This figure shows an example of an MRI.

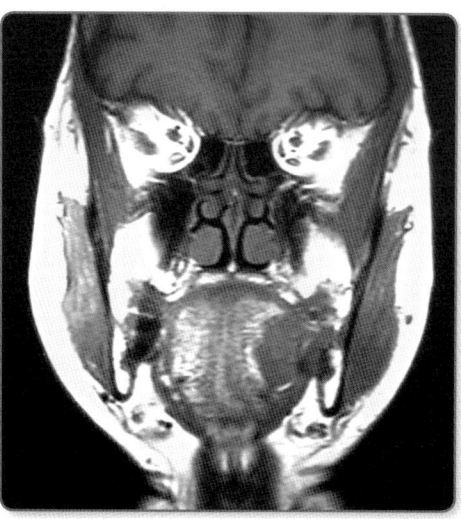

4.1 Question

How good is magnetic resonance (MR) imaging as demonstrated in this figure in assessing lymphadenopathy?

Answer

- MR is less operator-dependent than ultrasonography
- MR shows poorer sensitivity (64%), specificity (69%) and accuracy (66%) when staging the neck in oral squamous cell carcinoma compared to CT

4.2 Question

How can the performance of MR be improved?

Answer

- Diffusion-weighted MRI can increase sensitivity for metastatic lymph nodes to 98% and specificity as high as 97%
- Ultrasmall super-paramagnetic iron oxide (USPIO)-enhanced MRI improves diagnostic performance
- Short-tau inversion recovery (STIR) sequence enhances T2-weighted images by suppressing fat signal and highlighting tumoural tissue
- Valuable in difficult anatomic areas and diagnosing recurrence

4.3 Question
What is the role of MR in examining the primary tumour site?

Answer
- Will identify bony involvement of the mandible, upstaging oral tumours to T4 status and the extent of marrow involvement (Box A)
- Good at demonstrating perineural spread (e.g. palatine lesions, mandibular invasion) and involvement of pre-epiglottic fat in tongue base tumours, giving vital information about resectability

4.4 Question
How does oral cancer invade the mandible?

Answer
- This question has been dealt with comprehensively by Brown et al. in a series of publications (2003)
- There is no 'preferred' pattern of mandibular invasion, with the tumour invading wherever it abuts the mandible
- Rim resections should be angled obliquely to account for this
- Role of the inferior alveolar nerve as a pathway of invasion is overstated and an uncommon finding
- Bone involvement may be invasive/infiltrative or erosive/arrosive
- Invasive bone involvement is probably indicative of aggressive underlying tumour biology with increasing rates of associated nodal positivity and extracapsular spread

4.5 Question
Can MR be used to assess the neck?

Answer
- MR is equally sensitive as CT, and is commonly used when assessing a soft tissue oral cavity tumour
- Criteria for assessment are shown in Box B

Box A: Features suggestive of osseous involvement at the primary site on MR

- The following features are cited by Trotta et al. (2011) as being indicative of likely osseous involvement on MRI
- Loss of low-signal-intensity cortex
- Replacement of high-signal-intensity marrow on T1-weighted images by intermediate-signal-intensity tumour
- Contrast enhancement within bone
- Contrast enhancement of nerves, e.g. inferior alveolar nerve
- STIR sequences improve MR sensitivity to 97% in detecting mandibular involvement
- MR tends to over-estimate rate of mandibular invasion
- Clinical examination, periosteal stripping intraoperatively and complementary imaging techniques (e.g. CT and MRI) allow a confident final decision

> **Box B: MR criteria for lymph node involvement**
> - The Head and Neck Cancer Multidisciplinary Management Guidelines recommend that nodes >10 mm diameter be regarded as involved
> - The exception is the junctional nodes (e.g. jugulodigastric node) at 15 mm
> - Other criteria include maximum longitudinal/short axis diameter <2.0, spherical shape and groups of 3+ borderline nodes

Further reading

de Bree R, Takes RP, Castelijns JA, et al. Advances in diagnostic modalities to detect occult lymph node metastases in head and neck squamous cell carcinoma. Head Neck 2015; 37:1829–1839.

Stuckensen T, Kovács AF, Adams S, Baum RP. Staging of the neck in patients with oral cavity squamous cell carcinomas: a prospective comparison of PET, ultrasound, CT and MRI. J Craniomaxillofac Surg 2000; 28:319–324.

Short case 5: Ultrasound assessment of neck lumps

You have referred the patient shown in this figure for an ultrasound scan following their presentation with a slowly developing lump at the angle of their mandible.

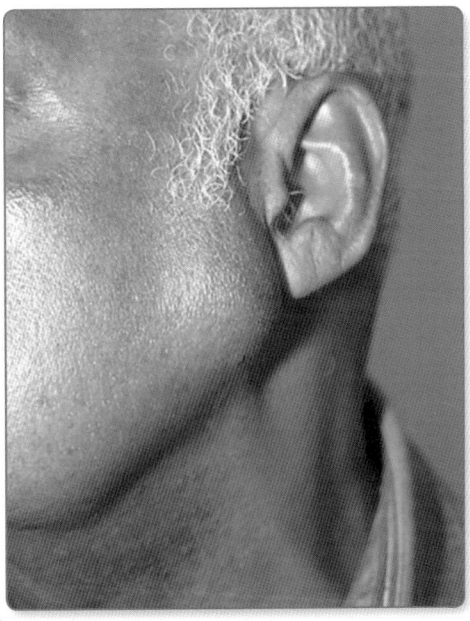

5.1 Question

How effective is ultrasonography in assessing cervical lymphadenopathy?

Answer

- Ultrasound combined with fine needle aspirate cytology (FNAC) has specificity of nearly 100% with few false positives
- Sensitivity highly variable (48–73%) with considerable operator dependence and heterogeneity in terms of identifying a lymph node worth sampling (Box A)
- Compared with other imaging modalities, US-FNAC often shows best performance in terms of accuracy (Box B)

5.2 Question

What does ultrasound add to a staging strategy with CT/MRI?

Answer

- Ultrasound decreases false-negative rate in staging patients as cN0
- This false negative rate in a treatment regimen with sentinel node where cN0 patients would be offered the service and only cN+ patients would undergo a selective neck dissection (SND)

- Norling et al. (2014) demonstrated that occult metastatic disease in the CT/MRI-staged N0 neck decreased from 31% to 18% with the addition of ultrasound

5.3 Question

What is the role of ultrasound in assessing salivary gland masses?

Answer

- Ultrasonography can correctly differentiate malignant lesions from benign ones in the salivary glands in 90% of cases and distinguish glandular from extraglandular masses in 98% of instances
- The facial nerve cannot be imaged, but its position inferred by examining intraglandular vessels
- Ultrasound is initial examination of choice in examining major salivary glands, which when combined with FNAC again results in high levels of accuracy

5.4 Question

What is the role of ultrasound in examining the thyroid?

Answer

- Ultrasound extremely sensitive for diagnosis of thyroid carcinoma, aiding decisions concerning appropriateness of FNAC
- Various criteria used to determine likelihood of malignancy including Kim Criteria, American Association of Clinical Endocrinologists Criteria and Society of Radiologists in Ultrasound
- Radiologists commonly ascribe U classification (U1–U5) in terms of likelihood of malignancy based on sonographic appearances (Box C)

Box A: Criteria for the suspicious node

- International criteria to discriminate between N0 and N+ necks on ultrasound findings are distinctly lacking
- Commonly used criteria include size, hypoechoic or heterogenous internal structure, irregular LN border, absence of hilum, spherical shape and peripheral nodal blood flow pattern
- The lower the cut-off point in terms of size for a suspicious node, the higher the sensitivity and the lower the specificity
- Norling et al. (2014) demonstrated that regarding 4 mm axial diameter as suspicious would give an 85.7% sensitivity and 38% specificity
- By comparison increasing this to 9 mm would yield a 100% specificity but 19% sensitivity. Short axial diameter is the most predictive feature according to Norling et al.
- US upstaged 14% of patients to N+ classed as cN0 by CT/MRI but also classified 6% as N+ who were subsequently shown to be pN0 following dissection
- Odds ratios are given for heterogenous appearance (1.2), irregular border (5.7), spherical shape (6.0), absence of nodal hilum (6.0) and peripheral nodal blood flow (5.2)

> **Box B: de Bondt et al. (2007) and diagnostic odds ratios**
> - de Bondt et al. carried out a meta-analysis in 2007 and calculated diagnostic odds ratios (DORs) for different imaging modalities in the detection of lymph node metastases
> - The DOR combines sensitivity and specificity into one measure
> - They demonstrated the highest DOR to be seen with USgFNAC which also demonstrated the highest specificity (98%)
> - Sensitivity was highest for US (87%) when compared with MRI, CT and USPIO-MRI (Sinerem)

> **Box C: the U classification used in ultrasound assessment**
> - U1–U2 lesions should not be subjected to FNAC, as this increases the chances of overtreatment of clinically insignificant micropapillary thyroid carcinomas (micro-PTCs)
> - U3–U5 subjected to FNAC with cytology results being given a Thy status (Thy1–Thy5)
> - These then determine ongoing treatment with the likelihood of malignancy increasing with the score
> - For example follicular or indeterminate cytology (Thy3) is followed by malignant histology in 9.5–43% of cases, while Thy 4 nodules prove to be malignant in 68–70% of instances

Further reading

Norling R, Buron BM, Therkildsen MH, et al. Staging of cervical lymph nodes in oral squamous cell carcinoma: adding ultrasound in clinically lymph node negative patients may improve diagnostic work-up. PLoS One 2014; 9:1–6.

Perros P, Boelaert K, Colley S, et al. Guidelines for the management of thyroid cancer. Clin Endocrin 2014; 81:1–122.

Short case 6: Unknown primary and PET scanning

This patient with suspected oral cancer has returned to clinic to discuss the results of this scan.

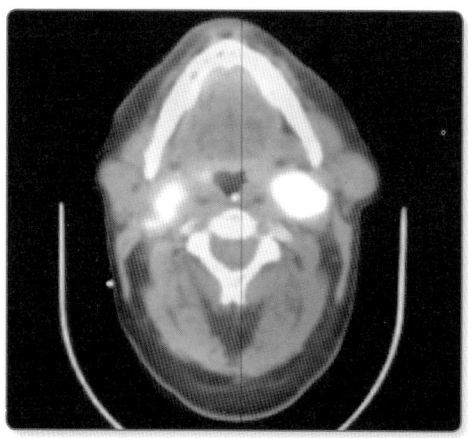

6.1 Question

How does cancer of the unknown primary present?

Answer

- Cancer of unknown primary (CUP) usually manifests as neck lump or lumps with no primary index site
- Will most commonly be level II or III
- Neck node location gives clues to location of a possible subclinical primary (e.g. a level I node would imply oral cavity whilst level VI would be more in keeping with thyroid, larynx or cervical oesophagus)

6.2 Question

What does cystic adenopathy imply?

Answer

- Cystic lymph node is hallmark of human papilloma virus (HPV)-associated adenopathy
- Usually from an undiagnosed oropharyngeal tumour, especially if metastatic squamous cell carcinoma (SCC) is identified on fine needle aspirate cytology (FNAC)

6.3 Question

How should CUP be investigated?

Answer

- Thorough clinical examination of upper aerodigestive tract including flexible nasendoscopy (FNE) and palpation the tongue base in particular, as well as cutaneous head and neck examination
- FNAC/core biopsy of any adenopathy
- Clues on pathology, e.g. Epstein–Barr virus (EBV) implying nasopharyngeal primary, HPV pointing to oropharyngeal disease
- Cross-sectional imaging (CT) skull base to diaphragm
- Low threshold for PET-CT to identify primary site or guide possible biopsies at panendoscopy (Box A)

6.4 Question

What if the PET-CT reveals no site?

Answer

- Panendoscopy and biopsy of anything suspicious as well as ipsilateral/bilateral tonsillectomy and/or 'targeted' biopsies of tongue base, postnasal space and/or pyriform fossa (Boxes B and C)
- If transoral robotic surgery (TORS) service in place, tongue base mucosectomy can be considered, but this still requires prospective evaluation

6.5 Question

What modifications of technique exist?

Answer

- Surgery alone (modified radical neck dissection) may be sufficient for N1 neck with no extracapsular spread (ECS)
- ECS or N2 stage or higher should prompt adjuvant treatment (chemo/radiotherapy). No conclusive evidence to support routine practice of total mucosal irradiation (TMI) with current national guidelines recommending this is at discretion of treating clinician

---

Box A: The PET-NECK Trial

- Previously, common practice following chemoradiotherapy for advanced nodal stage nodal disease head and neck cancer (N2–N3) was either planned neck dissection or image-guided surveillance
- This trial recruited 564 patients in a randomised controlled trial
- It demonstrated that PET-CT guided surveillance resulted in fewer neck dissections with similar complication rates, overall survival at 2 years (84.9% vs. 81.5%) and quality of life
- The PET-CT approach was more cost effective

> **Box B: NICE guidance on PET**
> - The National Institute for Health and Care Excellence (NICE) recommends consideration of a PET scan as the first line investigation in CUP with metastatic nodal SCC in order to identify a possible primary
> - In addition, PET scans are recommended for stating in T4 cancers of the hypopharynx or nasopharynx and any N3 cancers of the upper aerodigestive tract

> **Box C: PET-CT sensitivity**
> - CUP accounts for less than 5% of head and neck cancers
> - The PET-CT will establish a primary site in around one third of patients presenting as CUP
> - A 2009 systematic review and metanalysis revealed primary detection rate, sensitivity and specificity of 37%, 84% and 84% respectively
> - Combining this data with a separate paper from 2013, the UK National Multidisciplinary Guidelines give these figures as 44%, 97% and 68%

Further reading

Kwee TC, Kwee RM. Combined FDG-PET/CT for the detection of unknown primary tumours: systematic review and meta-analysis. Eur Radiol 2009; 19:731–744.

Mackenzie K, Watson M, Jankowska P, et al. Investigation and management of the unkown primary with metastatic neck disease: United Kingdom National Multidisciplinary Guidelines. J Laryngol Otol 2016; 130:S170–S175.

Mehanna H, Wong WL, McConkey CC, et al. The PET-CT surveillance versus neck dissection in advanced head and neck cancer. N Engl J Med 2016; 374:1444–1454.

National Institute for Health and Care Excellence. Cancer of the upper aerodigestive tract: assessment and management in people aged 16 and over. Clinical guideline NG36. London: NICE, 2016.

Short case 7: Sentinel lymph node biopsy

A patient with oral cancer is about to have an investigation using the items shown in this figure.

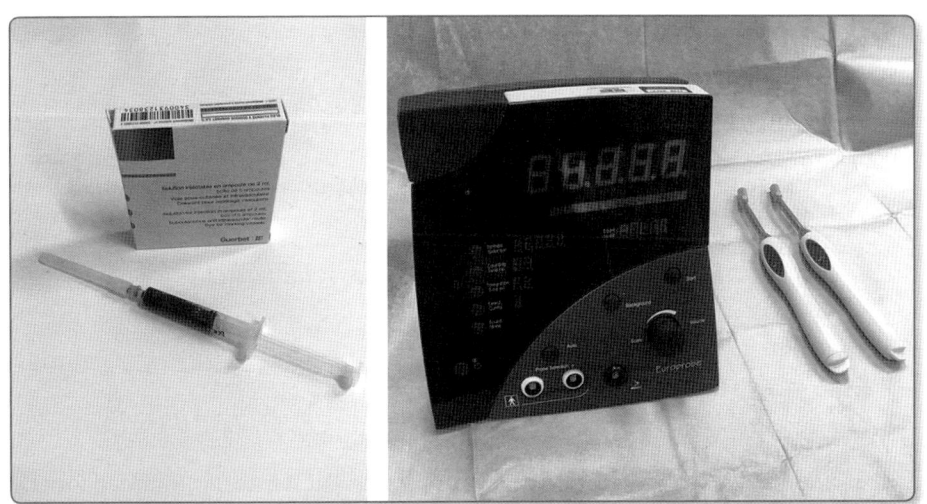

7.1 Question
What investigation is about to take place?

Answer

The patient is likely to be having sentinel lymph node biopsy (SNLB) of his neck.

7.2 Question
What might you expect to find on examining their neck?

Answer

- One or more scars placed along where a conventional neck dissection scar would be
- If performed recently, may be some blue dye at primary site still lingering

7.3 Question
How is SNLB performed?

Answer

- Patients are injected with radioactive tracer such as technetium 99 m either day before or on morning of surgery (Box A)
- Patients attend nuclear medicine department for lymphoscintigraphy
- At surgery, a hand-held gamma probe used to look for 'hot' nodes

- Placement of blue dye at primary site at start of surgery also colours the nodes to aid their localisation
- Counts taken of node and residuals following removal

7.4 Question

What are the risks of surgery specific to SNLB?

Answer

- Damage to adjacent structures (e.g. accessory nerve) as for any lymph node biopsy
- Allergic reaction to blue dye (<1/1000 cases)
- Patients should be aware that use of blue dye is unlicensed

7.5 Question

Who should be offered sentinel node biopsy?

Answer

- The NICE guidance from 2016 recommends SNLB is recommended for any patient with a T1–T2 N0 oral tumour who does not require neck access to facilitate reconstruction with free tissue transfer (Box B)

7.6 Question

What is the 'shine through' effect?

Answer

- Due to proximity of primary site to sentinel node, detection of the sentinel node with gamma probe may be compromised when angled towards primary site
- Particularly an issue in floor of mouth tumours where sensitivity found to fall from 94–97% to 80–86%

7.7 Question

What should patients be told?

Answer

- Like melanoma, as soon as sentinel node offers meaningful prognostic information
- SNB negative disease has statistically better overall survival
- FNRs as low as 7% have been seen and strategy may offer comparable outcomes to a more traditional treatment approach in terms of disease control and overall survival
- Significance of micrometastases and isolated tumour cells (ITCs) remains to be seen
- Role of completion lymphadenectomy and how extensive surgery will be need to be explained

Box A: The SENT trial

- A multinational prospective trial of 415 patients with T1–T2 N0 oral squamous cell carcinoma (SCC)
- Sentinel node biopsy (SNB) had a sensitivity of 86%
- Eighty five percent of those with a positive SNB had no positive non-sentinel node (NSN) on completion lymphadenectomy
- Of the 14% false negative rate (FNR) only half (53.3%) were amenable to salvage when they recurred
- Six percent of occult cervical metastases were contralateral
- Whilst the FNR rate was higher than desirable, this was operator dependent in their estimation and they cited a 'learning curve'
- The detrimental effect of the FNR was offset by the detection of contralateral disease, that a conventional treatment strategy (ipsilateral elective neck dissection) would have missed

Box B: Relevance of sentinel node sampling

- Traditionally the standard of neck dissection was set at a likelihood of 20% occult metastases in the N0 neck
- This meant that potentially 70–80% of patients with radiologically and clinically N0 necks are 'over treated'
- D'Cruz et al. published a landmark paper in 2015 that demonstrated a significant survival advantage in elective neck dissection versus therapeutic neck dissection at the point of recurrence for early oral SCC
- The paper hinted at the possibility that this may not hold true for thinner tumours (3 mm or less)
- Sentinel node may therefore offer comparable regional control whilst minimizing the morbidity of a full neck dissection

Further reading

De Bree R, Nieweg OE. The history of sentinel node biopsy in head and neck cancer: from visualization of lymphatic vessesl to sentinel nodes. Oral Oncol 2015; 51:819–23.

D'Cruz AK, Vaish R, Kapre N, et al. Elective versus therapeutic neck dissection in node negative oral cancer. N Engl J Med 2015; 373:521–529.

National Institute for Health and Care Excellence. Cancer of the upper aerodigestive tract: assessment and management in people aged 16 and over. NICE, 2016.

Schilling C, Stoeckli SJ, Haerle SK, et al. Sentinel European Node Trial (SENT): 3-year results of sentinel node biopsy in oral cancer. Eur J Cancer 2015; 51:2777–2784.

Short case 8: Oropharyngeal cancer

A patient has been referred for a suspicious lesion in their left tonsil region.

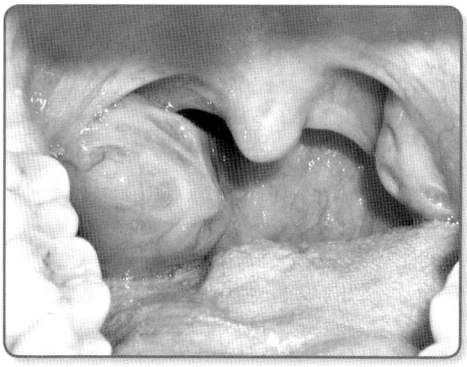

8.1 Question
How would you examine the primary site?

Answer

- Normal head and neck examination sequence
- Lip split mandibulotomy scars
- Neck dissection scars
- Osteoradionecrosis: mandibulotomy sites
- Stigmata of radiotherapy treatment
- Function and appearance of any reconstruction
- In reconstructions involving soft palate establish whether this is dynamic or static
- Degree of VPI: hypernasal speech, dysphagia

8.2 Question
How would you examine the nodal basins?

Answer

- Lymph node metastases from oropharyngeal cancers are predominantly levels II–IV
- Tonsilar SCC has a high preponderance of bilateral nodal involvement, which was 10% in the landmark paper by Woolgar et al.
- Tumours close to midline invite a low threshold for bilateral nodal dissections (conventionally IIs–IV +/– level Ib)

8.3 Question
What is the role of examination under anaesthesia (EUA) and panendoscopy?

Answer

- To establish extent and resectability of tumour

- Often only method of achieving tissue diagnosis
- Clinical staging of tumour, enabling treatment planning
- Serves as 'dry run' of patient's ability to tolerate general anaesthesia

8.4 Question

Should surgery be the treatment of choice for OPSCC?

Answer

- The Scottish Head and Neck Cancer audit (1999–2001) demonstrated no significant difference in disease-specific survival (DSS) for early stage disease when comparing surgical and nonsurgical treatments
- Radiotherapy effective in HPV positive cancers (Box C)
- The GETTEC study (Cosmidis et al. 2004) demonstrated 3-year OS rates of 95%
- With incidence of second primaries in head and neck region being 16–23%, adjuvant radiotherapy should arguably be held in reserve where possible
- Options for surgery are described in Boxes A and B

8.5 Question

What is the role of salvage surgery in recurrent OPSCC?

Answer

- Zafareo et al. (2009) found that salvage surgery conferred a 3-year OS rate of 48.7%
- Superior to reirradiation (2016 metanalysis by Jayaram et al.)
- Prognostic factors that impacted success of salvage surgery were age, disease-free interval and recurrent tumour stage

Box A: Transoral robotics and microsurgery

- The Veterans Affairs Laryngeal Cancer Study Group in 1991 showed statistically equivalent survival rates between surgery with adjuvant radiotherapy (RT) and induction chemotherapy followed by RT for laryngeal cancer patients
- This was extrapolated as the dogma of "organ preservation" for other head and neck subsites including the oropharynx
- Recently this has been challenged with the use of transoral robotic surgery (TORS) and transoral laser microsurgery (TLM)
- Rich et al. (2009) employed carbon dioxide TLM resection of stage III and IV oropharyngeal squamous cell carcinoma (OPSCC) +/− adjuvant treatment to demonstrate a 12% positive margin rate
- However this produced 2- and 5-year overall survival (OS) of 94% and 88% respectively with disease free survival rates (DFS) of 91% and 87% respectively
- TORS and TLM offer alternatives to the lip split mandibulotomy with its attendant morbidity and complications
- Transcervical pharyngotomy is another option for tongue base tumours

> **Box B: Electrochemotherapy (ECT): a novel treatment modality?**
>
> - ECT works by 'electroporation', essentially delivering an electrical current to make cells more porous
> - This makes them more receptive to systemically or locally administered chemotherapy agents (commonly bleomycin)
> - A partial tumour response of 59% and complete response of 38% was seen in a study published by Campana et al. (2014) of a patient cohort including OPSCC

> **Box C: DAHANCA and HPV**
>
> - The implication of HPV in OPSCC is discussed in Scenario 3.1
> - Lassen et al. in DAHANCA have reported at length about the higher sensitivity of HPV/p16 positive OPSCC to RT, an effect not felt in other head and neck subsites

Further reading

Campana L, Mali B, Sersa G, et al. Electrochemotherapy in non-melanoma head and neck cancers: a retrospective analysis of the treated cases. Br J Oral Maxillofac Surg 2014; 52:957–964.

Cosmidis A, Rame JP, Dassonville O, et al. T1-T2 oropharyngeal cancers treated with surgery alone. A GETTEC study. Eur Arch Otorhinolaryngol 2004; 261:276–281.

Jayaram SC, Muzaffar SJ, Ahmed I, et al. Efficacy, outcomes and complication rates of difference surgical and non-surgical treatment modalities for recurrent/residual oropharyngeal carcinoma. Head Neck 2016; 38:1855–1861.

Woolgar J. The topography of cervical lymph node metastases revisited. Int J Oral Maxillofac Surg 2007; 36:219–225.

Short case 9: Radial forearm flap

A patient with recently treated oral cancer returns for follow up.

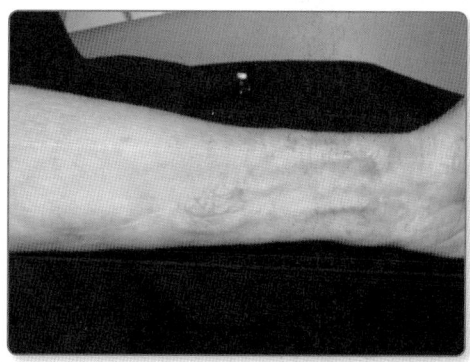

9.1 Question

What are the key features when examining the patient shown in the figure?

Answer

- Location of defect and type of flap used: fasciocutaneous, osteocutaneous
- If endosseus implants check these are successfully prosthodontically rehabilitated
- Donor site and morbidity: check whether full or split thickness skin graft and if sensory loss to dorsum of hand/first web space

9.2 Question

What are the advantages of the radial forearm flap?

Answer

- Soft tissue radial forearm flap a relatively straightforward dissection
- Good caliber vessels (particularly if cephalic vein harvested also)
- Predictable anatomy
- Provides supple thin skin, often regardless of patient's general habitus
- Allows for two-team approach to ablative and reconstructive surgery
- Can potentially harvest bone (Box A)

9.3 Question

What are the disadvantages?

Answer

- Skin often hair bearing
- Donor site can be unsightly and scar prone to contracture, particularly if split thickness skin graft used (Box C)
- Dorsal branch of the radial nerve at risk in dissection, resulting in persistent numbness of dorsal hand (1st web space)

9.4 Question

What are the indications?

Answer

- Being a very pliable flap, the radial forearm lends itself to anywhere that requires supple, mobile tissue, such as the floor of mouth, lateral tongue and buccal mucosa
- The composite radial is favoured by some for low-level maxillectomy defects
- The success rate for osseointegrated implants, however, is regarded as poor when compared with other composite free tissue transfer options such as the fibula (reported as low as 21% in a comparative study by Moscoso et al. 1994)
- The composite radial is also good for reconstruction of Brown class VI defects when used in combination with a paramedian forehead flap, with the skin from the radial flap acting as nasal lining

9.5 Question

What modifications of technique exist?

Answer

- Various design modifications have been employed, including changes to the shape of the skin paddle such as the bilobed, longitudinal, omega, beavertail and rectangular template techniques (Box B)
- Modifications to the dissection include raising the flap as a supra-fascial dissection and closing the donor site with ulnar flaps, Z-plasties, bilobed flaps or V-Y advancement flaps to avoid skin grafts
- Adipofascial flaps can be harvested to allow skin to close primarily and tissue expanders
- Minor modifications such as de-epithelialisation allow for optimal aesthetics at the commissure (Elledge et al. 2017)

Box A: Fractures and the composite radial forearm flap

- The incidence of fracture at the donor site for composite radial flaps was reported to be in the region of 15–25%
- Avery (2013) did work on finite element analysis (FEA) of the donor site
- This demonstrated that differing types of osteotomy cuts may reduce stress levels by 56%
- When coupled with prophylactic plating with a 3.5 mm steel dynamic compression plate (DCP) such measures lessen the likelihood of fracture considerably
- No >25% of the circumference of the radius should be harvested

Box B: Nerves, veins and tendons

- Harvesting the cephalic vein yields a diameter that is much larger than the venae comitantes that run with the artery (3 mm vs. 1.5 mm)
- The lateral or medial cutaneous nerves of the forearm may be harvested where a sensate flap is required
- The palmaris longus tendon may be used in areas such as recreating the oral sphincter

Box C: Challengers for 'workhorse' status

- In recent years a growing number of flaps have challenged the radial forearm flap's status as the 'workhorse' flap of maxillofacial surgery
- The medial sural artery perforator (MSAP) flap offers minimal donor site morbidity in comparison
- The perforator anterolateral thigh (ALT) flap is also a contender
- Both of these are more technically demanding dissections
- The ALT in Western populations often is significantly bulkier, requiring aggressive thinning either at the time of insetting or subsequently
- The MSAP flap may have unpredictability and inconsistency in terms of the number and location of perforators and the donor site cannot always be closed primarily
- The radial forearm flap may yet hold its status

Further reading

Avery CME. Review of the radial free flap: is it still evolving or is it facing extinction? Part one: soft tissue radial flap. Br J Oral Maxillofac Surg 2010; 48:245–252.

Moscoso JF, Keller J, Genden E, et al. Vascularized bone flaps in oromandibular reconstruction. A comparative anatomic study of bone stock from various donor sites to assess for suitability for endosseus dental implants. Arch Otolaryngol Head Neck Surg 1994; 120:36–43.

Short case 10: Fibula flap

This patient is returning for follow up at a year post surgery and reconstruction for oral cancer.

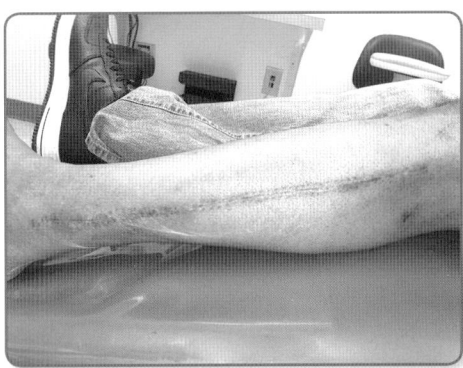

10.1 Question

What are the key features to be aware of when examining the patient shown in the above figure?

Answer

- Classify location of defect (Box A)
- Determine type of flap used: skin paddle present, single segment or multiple osteotomies, double-barreled
- Endosseus implants and prosthodontic rehabilitation
- Donor site and morbidity: whether full or split thickness skin graft
- Foot drop or sensory deficit

10.2 Question

What are the advantages of the fibula flap?

Answer

- The fibula flap provides good length of bone (up to 26 cm)
- Tolerates multiple osteotomies well and supports endosseus implants
- Donor site can often be closed primarily up to a width of 6 cm and the pedicle length is good

10.3 Question

What are the disadvantages of the fibula flap?

Answer

- Skin paddle: often hair bearing and depends on perforators which can make it unreliable

- Common peroneal nerve: at risk proximally during dissection and foot drop a recognised complication
- This is more commonly due to pressure from backslabs
- Lower limb vessels more prone to atherosclerosis making microvascular anastomoses challenging, or precluding use of fibula all together
- Risk of compartment syndrome (Box B)

10.4 Question

What investigations should be requested?

Answer

- Doppler ultrasonography of the lower limb ensures adequate supply from the anterior and posterior tibial vessels to permit harvesting of peroneal vessels
- Anatomical variations exist (Box C)
- MR angiogram (MRA) less operator dependent
- Computed tomography angiography (CTA) allows manipulation of DICOM data for surgical planning and custom cutting guides

10.5 Question

What are the indications for use?

Answer

- Fibula lends itself to segmental mandibular defects
- Ideal for total mandibulectomy defects due to its ability to tolerate multiple osteotomy sites
- Also used for low level (class II) maxillectomy defects or more challenging maxillary reconstructions when 'folded' on itself at interspersed osteotomy sites

10.6 Question

How successful are implants placed in fibulas?

Answer

- Studies quote implant survival rates of 93% and successful prosthodontic rehabilitation of surviving implants as high as 98%
- Compromise is between height of implant in relation to native dentition and need to restore contour of lower border
- Measures to improve success include placing the fibula "midway" between lower border and ideal alveolar ridge height or "double-barreling" the reconstruction

> **Box A: Classification of segmental mandibular defects**
> - The most widely recognised is that developed by James Brown et al. (2016)
> - The mandible is effectively divided into quadrants by the four "corners" of the two angles and two canines
> - Lateral defect (not including canine)
> - Hemimandibulectomy (involving ipsilateral canine)
> - Anterior (including both canines)
> - Extensive (including canines and angles)
> - The suffix "c" is then added to denote whether or not the condyle is also sacrificed
> - The Boyd system (1993) is similar in using "H", "L" and "C" denoting the extent of resection based on involvement of condyles and canines
> - Suffices "o", "s", "m" and "sm" describe whether or not skin and/or oral mucosa is sacrificed

> **Box B: Compartment syndrome and the free fibula flap**
> - Compartment syndrome is a potentially limb-threatening complication
> - Whilst compartment pressures can be measured, clinical suspicion should prompt a low threshold for surgical re-exploration
> - As all fascial compartments have been explored in raising the flap, a formal fasciotomy is not required

> **Box C: Arterial anatomical variants**
> - Peroneal arteria magna: where the peroneal is the dominant supply to the foot (8%)
> - Complete absence: 0.1%

Further reading

Brown JS, Barry C, Ho M, Shaw R, et al. A new classification for mandibular defects after oncological resection. Lancet Oncol 2016; 17:e23–30.

Jackson RS, Price DL, Arce K, Moore EJ, et al. Evaluation of clinical outcomes of osseointegrated dental implantation of fibula free flaps. JAMA Facial Plast Surg 2016; 18:201–206.

Kerrary S, Schouman T, Cox A, et al. Acute compartment syndrome following fibula flap harvest for mandibular reconstruction. J Craniomaxillofac Surg 2011; 39:206–208.

Salgado CJ, et al. Fibula flap. In: Wei F-C, Mardini S (Eds), Flaps and Reconstructive Surgery Elsevier Saunders, 2009.

Short case 11: Pectoralis major myocutaneous flap

This patient has returned to clinic following the surgical procedure shown in the figure below.

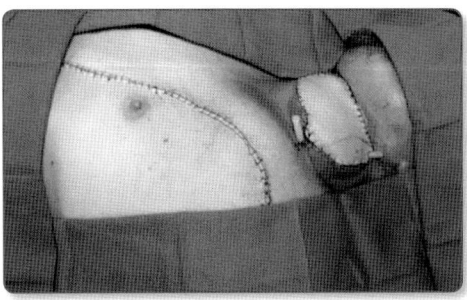

11.1 Question

What are the key features to be aware of when examining the patient shown in this figure?

Answer

- Location of defect and whether tunneled or muscle pedicle grafted (Box A)
- Muscle only or skin island included
- Use of a 'defensive' incision (Box B)

11.2 Question

What are the vessel(s) supplying the flap?

Answer

- Clavicular and pectoral heads of the thoracoacromial artery are the dominant supply to the muscle
- Minor contributions come from internal mammary artery (IMA) perforators, intercostal artery perforators and pectoral branch of lateral thoracic artery

11.3 Question

What are the advantages of the PMMC flap?

Answer

- The PMMC flap is relatively easy to harvest with consistent anatomy and short operating time
- As pedicled flap outside radiotherapy field, it is viable alternative to free tissue transfer in irradiated and/or vessel-depleted neck

11.4 Question

What are the disadvantages?

Answer

- Distortion of chest wall and unaesthetic appearance
- Limited arc of rotation and distance
- Excessive bulk
- Chest wall haematomas/infections
- Partial necrosis of skin paddle (up to 12%)

11.5 Question

What modifications do you know?

Answer

- Vascularised bone incorporated, e.g. rib
- Nerve inclusion to achieve dynamic muscle action
- Double paddle flap incorporating throracoacromial and lateral thoracic arteries
- Extended parasternal paddle using contralateral internal mammary perforators
- Muscle free pedicle
- Feasibility of subclavicular route to lengthen pedicle and improve mobility

11.6 Question

What are the indications for use?

Answer

- Carotid artery protection after radical neck dissection
- Cervical skin defects
- Dead space filler, e.g. salvage laryngectomies
- Vessel depleted necks
- Mandible reconstruction following previous free flap failure or when free tissue transfer not advisable (a poor substitute)
- Pharyngocutaneous fistulae
- Partial (<50% circumferential) laryngectomies

Box A: Pedicled flaps used in head and neck reconstruction

- With an ageing population surviving longer with challenging comorbidities, pedicled flaps may be making something of a comeback
- Be aware of the following options in head and neck reconstruction
- Pectoralis major myocutaneous (PMMC) flap
- Submental island flap
- Temporalis/temporoparietal fascia (TPF) flap
- Facial artery musculomucosal (FAMM) flap
- Supraclavicular flap
- Trapezius flap
- Deltopectoral flap
- Internal mammary artery perforator (IMAP) flap

Box B: The deltopectoral flap

- Whilst the PMMC may be seen as a back-up plan in its own right, the deltopectoral (DP) flap is the PMMC's back up
- Whilst some incorporate into a "defensive" incision when raising the PMMC, preserving the intercostals at the time of raising the PMMC is sufficient to maintain the option of a later DP
- It is based on parasternal fasciocutaneous perforating branches of the IMA but has a high distal flap necrosis rate (10–25%)
- The IMA may be needed for bypass grafting so its use should be guarded in patients with ischaemic heart disease

Further reading

Bussu F, Gallus R, Navach V, et al. Contemporary role of pectoralis major regional flaps in head and neck surgery. Acta Otorhinolaryngol Ital 2014; 34:327–341.

Hsing CY, Wong YK, Wang CP, et al. Comparison between free flap and pectoralis major pedicled flap for reconstruction in oral cavity cancer patients – a quality of life analysis. Oral Oncol 2011; 47:522–527.

Kingdom T, Singer M. Enhanced reliability and renewed applications of the deltopectoral flap in head and neck reconstruction. Laryngoscope 1996; 106:1230–1233.

Short case 12: Anterolateral thigh flap

This patient returns to clinic following suture removal from his leg surgical site.

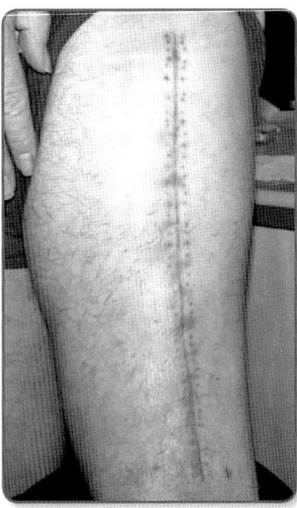

12.1 Question

What are the key features to be aware when examining the patient shown in this figure?

Answer

- Location of defect and type of flap used (e.g. de-epithelialised)
- Donor site morbidity, e.g. need for skin graft, sensory deficit lateral thigh

12.2 Question

What are the advantages of the anterolateral thigh (ALT) flap?

Answer

- ALT flap provides relatively constant anatomy, long length and a large pedicle
- Donor site can be closed primarily up to width of 7–9 cm and flaps can be sensate
- Flap harvest can be performed concurrent with resection and variability in design means potential for bulk (with vastus lateralis) or pliability (as thinned perforator flap)

12.3 Question

What are the disadvantages of an ALT flap?

Answer

- Skin may be a poor colour match for head and neck

- Occasionally donor site requires grafting which can be unsightly
- Sensory loss to lateral thigh not uncommon, although prevented by suprafascial dissection

12.4 Question

What are the indications for an ALT flap?

Answer

- Pliable and supple when raised as a perforator flap
- Good for resurfacing intraoral defects as well as larger cutaneous defects around head and neck that would preclude local flap repair
- Conversely, when raised with vastus lateralis (perforators not formally chased in the dissection), provides bulk which may enable reconstruction of larger glossectomy defects with a static reconstruction
- Tubed ALT flaps have been used for reconstruction in parastomal recurrence after total laryngectomy; tubed flaps also find a role in laryngopharynectomy reconstruction (Box A)
- ALT also good for relining Brown class V maxillectomy defects, as allows sufficient thinning to create the hollow contour necessary to take an orbital prosthesis (Box B)
- Class I defects can also be repaired with the fat and soft tissue bulk filling dead space and reducing the chance of dehiscence

12.5 Question

What modifications of ALT flap technique exist?

Answer

- Chimeric flap: uses separate skin paddles based on different perforators when raised as true perforator flap (enables simultaneous resurfacing of intra- and extraoral defects)
- Vascularised iliac bone
- Vascularised fibula bone
- Flaps can be thinned aggressively (Box C) to generate more pliable soft tissue profile

---

Box A: Flap thinning

- Flap thinning may be performed by "conventional" technique of secondary removal of adipose tissue after raising a a full-thickness flap
- The other option is microdissection by dissection of blood vessels in the adipose layer under the operative microscope. The flap can be thinned to 3 mm provided the flap is within 9 cm of the perforator

> **Box B: Classification systems**
> - Mathes and Nahai classify cutaneous flaps by fascial perforators as type A (direct cutaneous), B (septocutaneous) or C (musculocutaneous)
> - Nakajima et al., give a more detailed breakdown as: I direct cutaneous; II septocutaneous; III perforating cutaneous branch of muscular vessel; IV direct cutaneous branch of muscular vessel; V septocutaneous perforator; VI musculocutaneous perforator
> - Cormack and McCarthy provide another system. You should also know classifications for muscular flaps (e.g. Taylor) and bony flaps (e.g. Serafin)

> **Box C: Laryngopharyngectomy**
> - Pharyngeal defects can be reconstructed with tubed radial forearm, ALT, gastro-omental flaps or free jejunal flaps
> - Whilst cutaneous flaps are thought to give superior outcomes in terms of speech rehabilitation (the jejunal flaps producing a "wet" voice), swallowing is thought to be better with jejunum
> - Flap survival of jejunum in a series in Birmingham was 97% with 91% of patients able to resume an oral diet on discharge, 73% maintaining oral diet at 3 years and 70% using their voice in everyday situations

Further reading

Brown JS, Shaw RJ. Reconstruction of the maxilla and midface: introducing a new classification. Lancet Oncol 2010; 11:1001–1008.

Chim H, Salgado CJ, Seselgyte R, et al. Principles of head and neck reconstruction: an algorithm to guide flap selection. Semin Plast Surg 2010; 24:148–154.

Mardini S, et al. Anterolateral thigh flap. In: Wei F-C, Mardini S (Eds) Flaps and Reconstructive Surgery Elsevier Saunders, 2009.

Walker RJ, Parmar S, Praveen P, et al. Jejunal free flap for reconstruction of pharyngeal defects in patients with head and neck cancer: the Birmingham experience. Br J Oral Maxillofac Surg 2014; 52:106–110.

Short case 13: Scapular flap

This patient is being prepared for reconstruction for a planned oncological resection.

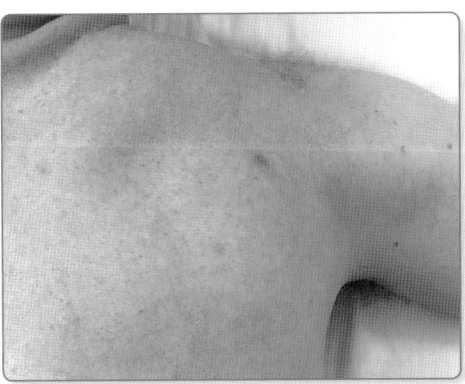

13.1 Question
What are the key features to be aware of when examining the patient shown in this figure?

Answer
- Examine donor site scar and orientation (e.g. scapular or parascapular)
- Confirm if osseocutanous or soft tissue only
- Check for endosseus implants and if successfully prosthodontically rehabilitated
- Donor site and morbidity: full or split thickness skin graft

13.2 Question
What are the advantages of the scapular/parascapular flap?

Answer
- Generous amounts of soft tissue on consistent and reliable pedicle
- Minimal/no functional morbidity at donor site
- Colour match often superior in comparison to other flaps when reconstructing head and neck defects
- Lends itself to chimeric flaps with different designs possible around scapular axis and various vessels from circumflex scapular artery (Box A)
- Good success rates (Box B)

13.3 Question
What are the disadvantages of the scapular/parascapular flap?

Answer
- Patients must be positioned lateral decubitus or prone prolonging operative time and prohibiting two-team concurrent operating for most head and neck defects

- Sensory reinnervation not possible
- Large flaps mean difficulty in closing donor site and potential need for skin grafting

13.4 Question

What are the indications for the scapular/para-scapular flap?

Answer

- Scapular flap lends itself to maxillary reconstruction
- TDAA flap yields latissimus dorsi in chimeric fashion and bone capable of reliably supporting osseointegrated implants
- TDAA flap used by Brown and Shaw for class III and IV maxillectomy defects
- Facilitates mandibulectomy defects where extensive soft tissue bulk required, e.g. anterior glossectomies and retromolar trigone/oropharynx where contracture liable to invite velopharyngeal incompetence

13.5 Question

What modifications of technique exist?

Answer

- Various design modifications are possible (Box A)
- Classic horizontal incision based on transverse branch of CSA yields scapular flap, while skin paddle angled downwards based on descending branch gives parascapular flap
- Ascending vertical flap and inframammary extended circumflex scapular flap (IMECC)
- Scapular tip can be harvested on thoracodorsal angular artery (TDAA) and lends itself to maxillary reconstruction

---

Box A: Vascular anatomy

- The axillary artery gives the subscapular artery, which in turn divides into the thoracodorsal artery (TDAP/TDAA flap) and circumflex scapular artery (scapular/parascapular flaps)
- The superficial branch of the CSA passes out through the triangular space between the triceps and two teres muscles to give the vertical/descending branch (parascapular flap) and the horizontal/transverse branch (scapular flap)
- The former forms a vascular arcade with the TDAP and the latter with the medial intercostals
- The main trunk of the CSA gives a descending branch that runs along the lateral border of the scapula to supply it, a branch to teres minor, a branch to teres major, a branch to infraspinatus, the terminal branch to the subscapularis and the cutaneous branch
- In this way, the flaps around the scapular axis have the potential to be true chimeric flaps with a range of options for design to include skin, muscle and bone

> **Box B: Success rates**
> - A review of flaps from Birmingham of the subscapular axis over a 16-year demonstrated a 6.4% failure rate
> - Brown et al. (2010) reported their results of 46 consecutive cases and had no absolute flap failures, but lost the bony component of the flap in 2/46 cases

Further reading

Angrigiani C, et al. Scapular and parascapular flaps. In: Wei F-C, Mardini S (Eds). Flaps and Reconstructive Surgery Elsevier Saunders, 2009.

Brown J, Bekiroglu F, Shaw R, et al. Indications for the scapular flap in reconstructions of the head and neck. Br J Oral Maxillofac Surg 2010; 48:331–337.

Siebert JW, Longaker MT, Angrigiani C. The inframammary extended circumflex scapular flap: an aesthetic improvement of the parascapular flap. Plast Reconstr Surg 1997; 99:70–77.

Young R, et al. Myo-osseus scapular flaps: the Birmingham experience. Br J Oral Maxillofac Surg 2016; 54: e170–e171.

Short case 14: Neck dissection

This patient returns to clinic for surveillance following surgery a year ago.

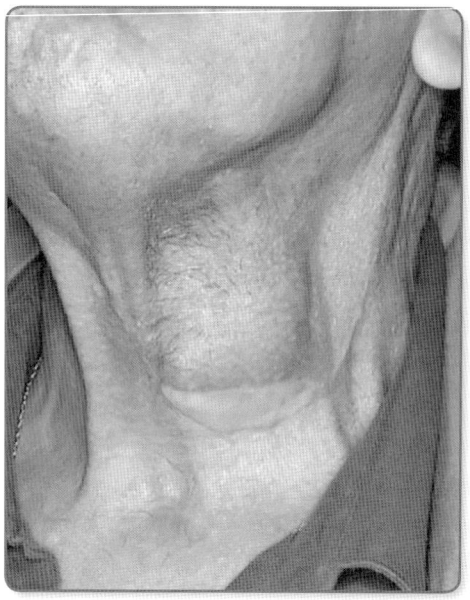

14.1 Question

What are the key features to be aware of when examining the patient shown in this figure?

Answer

- Neck dissection scars – be aware of different types, e.g. Crile's, MacFee
- Hallmarks of radiotherapy (e.g. skin changes)
- Palpate sternocleidomastoid to see if harvested
- Complications

14.2 Question

What are the possible complications?

Answer

- Shoulder weakness/stiffness
- Marginal mandibular nerve weakness (depressor anguli oris)
- Tongue numbness
- Chyle leak (Box A)
- Bleeding

14.3 Question
What are the indications for a neck dissection?

Answer
- Neck dissections can broadly be grouped as elective (N0) and therapeutic (N1)

14.4 Question
What are the staging investigations for the neck?

Answer
- Cross-sectional imaging required, either magnetic resonance imaging (MRI) or computer tomography (CT)
- Meta-analysis of imaging by de Bondt et al. (2007) showed mean sensitivity highest for ultrasonography (US) in diagnosing metastatic disease (87%)
- CT/MRI show lower interobserver variation and less operator-dependent performance

14.5 Question
When would you undertake an elective neck dissection?

Answer
- Traditionally threshold set at 20% likelihood of occult metastases, recognising that 70–80% of neck dissections were performed unnecessarily
- Recently this has been challenged with arrival of sentinel node, the Tata Memorial paper, superselective neck dissections and different follow-up strategies among other developments
- D'Cruz et al., compared elective neck dissection (END) with therapeutic neck dissection (TND) in early (T1–T2) oral cancer (Box B)

14.6 Question
Do you routinely dissect level 2B?

Answer
- This remains highly controversial but there is a growing trend towards performing it (Box C)

14.7 Question
Who should be offered adjuvant treatment?

Answer
- Two studies (EORTC #22931 and RTOG #9501) collated in comparative analysis by Bernier et al., (Box D)
- Presence of extracapsular spread (ECS) or positive margins should prompt consideration of chemoradiotherapy
- Presence of multiple nodes (pN2/pN3) or disease level IV or V are criteria for adjuvant radiotherapy

14.8 Question

When do you decide if a tumour is inoperable?

Answer
- Different surgeons (and different patients) have contrasting viewpoints on inoperability
- Sacrificing both IJVs should not be undertaken lightly and is reported to cause amaurosis
- Carotid artery is replaceable with interpositional graft
- Imaging features can provide a clue to inoperability around the carotid
- including 270° circumferential involvement, fascial plane deletion and an undefined wall)

Box A: Chyle leak management

- If identified intraoperatively, ligation under loupe magnification, local muscle flaps (e.g. sternocleidomastoid) and/or fibrin/cyanoacrylate glue may be used
- Low output leaks <1 L/day may be addressed by medium-chain triglyceride (MCT) or fat-free diet, with somatostatin/octreotide also being employed
- High output or refractory leaks require either sclerosants, lymphangiography-guided embolisation, endoscopic thoracic surgery
- Re-exploration of the wound is often a last resort

Box B: The Tata Memorial paper

- Enrollment was stopped early in this study by d'Cruz et al. due to superior results of END in terms of overall survival and disease-free survival
- There was a suggestion however that tumours <3 mm in thickness may not show a difference in outcomes between the two strategies

---

Box C: What is the value of dissecting level IIB routinely?

- The largest study by Lim et al. (2004) of 74 patients found 5.4% of patients had IIB involvement with no incidences of isolated level IIB without involvement of other lymph nodes in the supraomohyoid neck
- Similarly, a metanalysis by Lae et al. (2010) revealed 6.04% rate of IIB involvement in N0 necks
- Other studies including Pantvaidya et al. (2014) and Maher and Hoffman (2014) have shown the largest cohort of IIB positivity in tongue/retromolar trigone tumours
- This has led to some to call for restricting IIB dissection to these groups

Further reading

Bernier J, Cooper JS, Pajak TF, et al. Defining risk levels in locally advanced head and neck cancers Head Neck 2005; 27:843–850.

D'Cruz AK, Dandekar M, Vaish R, et al. Elective versus therapeutic neck dissection in node negative oral cancer. N Engl J Med 2015; 373:521–529.

Pantvaidya GH, Pal P, Vaidya AD, et al. Prospective study of 583 neck dissections in oral cancers: implications for clinical practice. Head Neck 2014; 36:1503–1507.

Short case 15: Upper lip defect reconstruction

This patient presents to your clinic immediately prior to surgery with his family for consenting.

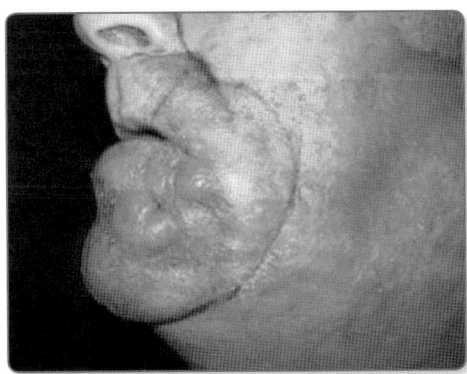

15.1 Question

What are the key features to be aware of when examining the patient shown in this figure?

Answer

- Determine whether competence of oral sphincter (orbicularis oris) maintained
- Whether vermillion border re-established
- Any microstomia
- Any sequelae to periodontal health
- Any sensory loss
- Any evidence of local recurrence
- Any cervical lymphadenopathy

15.2 Question

What are the indications for an Abbe flap?

Answer

- Abbe flap involves switching skin and vermillion from lower lip to upper lip (or vice versa) pedicled on labial artery
- Good for moderate length full thickness defects not involving commissure
- Frequently designed half size of defect to be reconstructed, thereby sharing the deficit between the two lips
- Pedicle requires division at second stage and patient motivation is key in intervening period

15.3 Question
What would you do about the commissure?

Answer
- This can be managed with an Abbe-Estlander flap, whereby tissue is switched between lips
- This is single stage surgery, as no pedicle has to be divided

15.4 Question
How would you manage a larger defect?

Answer
- Defects up to three-quarters length of lip may be treated with either perialar crescentic advancement flap (Burow-Diffenbach) or Karapndzic flap
- The Karapndzic flap taken down to muscle periorally but preserves motor supply to orbicularis oris muscle and sensory supply to overlying skin
- Extensive defects addressed with combined flaps such as bilateral melolabial (nasolabial) flaps and Abbe flap for philtrum
- Both flaps have the advantage of being hair bearing in male patients

15.5 Question
What options exist for restoring the vermillion?

Answer
- Smaller defects can be managed with mucosal advancement flaps
- Mucosal advancement flaps have drawback of contracting with healing and causing a thinner lip, and are best reserved for defects in vermillion remote from border/white roll
- Larger defects have been treated with superiorly based (reverse flow) facial artery myomucosal (FAMM) flap
- Vermillion switch procedures are useful
- Tongue flaps require patient compliance prior to pedicle division

---

Box A: Staging of lip tumours
- Lip tumours are most commonly squamous cell carcinomas (SCCs)
- They are staged along similar lines to the oral cavity
- They are slightly different to the remainder of the oral cavity in their approach and treatment
- Early stage malignancies (T1 and T2 N0) do not require cross-sectional imaging as part of their work-up routinely
- Radiotherapy (which may be external beam – EBRT – or brachytherapy) has comparable outcomes to surgery in terms of 5-year disease free survival and should be considered as a primary treatment modality

> **Box B: Epidemiology**
>
> - Cancers of the vermillion are best regarded as cutaneous malignancies
> - Incidence for this subsite is the commonest in the head and neck at 12/100 000
> - Solar radiation is the main risk factor

> **Box C: Greater than 80% length defects in the upper lip**
>
> - For such extensive defects, conventional local flap repairs will result in unacceptable degrees of microstomia
> - In such instances, recruiting nonlip skin becomes warranted in techniques such as the Webster-Barnard, McGregor and Nakajima
> - Free flaps such as the radial forearm are also reconstructive options
> - This may be a composite reconstruction in the case of an upper lip defect combined with an anterior maxillectomy
> - Finally, one should not forget maxillofacial prosthetic options, particularly in central defects combined with total or partial rhinectomy

Further reading

Baker SR. Local Flaps in Facial Reconstruction, Chapter 17. Reconstruction of the Lips, 3rd Edition. Elsevier, 2014.

Ferrari S, Ferri A, Bianchi B, et al. Head and neck reconstruction using the superiorly based reverse flow facial artery myomucosal flap. J Oral Maxillofac Surg 2015; 73:1008–1015.

Kerawala C, Roques T, Jeannon JP, Bisase B. Oral cavity and lip cancer: United Kingdom National Multidisciplinary Guidelines. J Laryngol Otol 2016; 130:S83–S89.

Short case 16: Radiotherapy

This patient has recently completed radiotherapy and returns to clinic for surveillance.

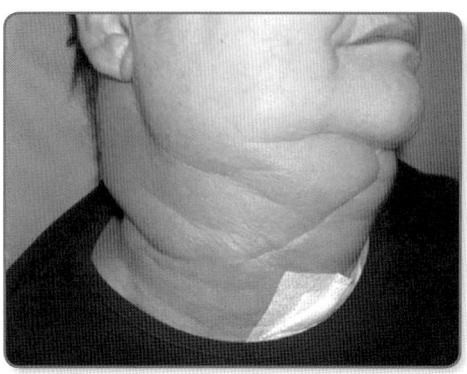

16.1 Question
What is the role of radiotherapy in relation to the patient shown in this figure?

Answer
- Early stage oral and oropharyngeal tumours show comparable outcomes with surgery or radiotherapy, albeit with different side-effect profile (Box A)
- Radiotherapy is used as an adjuvant treatment for N2+ neck and in combination with chemotherapy for involved margins and extracapsular spread (Box A)

16.2 Question
What are the recent advances in radiotherapy?

Answer
- Intensity-modulated radiotherapy (IMRT): computer-controlled linear accelerators used to deliver precise radiation doses to malignant tumor or specific areas within tumor
- Accelerated regimens: delivery of radiation over shorter time period
- Hyperfractionation: a higher dose delivered in multiple low-dose fractionations/day
- Drive to achieve comparable or superior local control with lower side-effect profiles

16.3 Question
What are radiosensitisers?

Answer
- Radiosensitisers are new drugs given to increase the efficacy of radiotherapy

- Examples include AT-101 (anti-Bcl-2), RAD001 (mTOR inhibitor), axitinib (VEGF inhibitor), bortezomib (anti-NF-kB) and GPI-15427 (poly-ADP-ribose polymerase inhibitor) among others
- Have been the subject of notable trials such as NIMRAD trial which compared nimorazole with placebo given concurrently with radiotherapy on back of evidence from DAHANCA5 in 1990s demonstrating improved locoregional control (49% vs. 33% at 5 years, $p = 0.002$)

16.4 Question

What are the stigmata of radiotherapy?

Answer

- Notable stigmata include mucositis, skin changes, xerostomia, caries, trismus and later osteoradionecrosis
- Radiotherapy not only decreases salivary flow, but alters composition [Moller et al. (2004) demonstrated decreased buffering capacity to 67%]

16.5 Question

How do you grade xerostomia?

Answer

- Xerostomia quantified using toxicity criteria (Box B)
- Criteria provided by Radiation Therapy Oncology Group and European Organisation for Research and Treatment of Cancer (RTOG/EORTC)

16.6 Question

What are the treatments for xerostomia?

Answer

- Stimulatory drugs: sugar-free gum, parasympathomimetics such as pilocarpine, good hydration
- Replacement drugs: sprays such as Glandosane

Box A: The evidence base behind radiotherapy

- MACH-NC (Pignon et al. 2009): A meta-analysis including 93 randomised trials and 17,346 patients, which demonstrated an absolute benefit of chemotherapy of 6.5% at 5 years when given concomitantly with radiotherapy in locally advanced head and neck cancer (LAHNCs)
- MARCH collaborative (Boorhis et al. 2006): Altered fractionation radiotherapy associated with an absolute survival benefit of 3.4%, increasing to 8% for hyperfractionated radiotherapy
- EORC 22931 and RTOG 9501 (Bernier et al. 2005): Combining chemotherapy with radiotherapy has benefits demonstrated in patients with ECS, positive histological margins (R1) or both. The survival benefits of chemotherapy are only felt in patients under 70 years of age

> **Box B: The PARSPORT trial and reducing xerostomia**
> - Nutting et al. (2011) reported a phase III randomised trial
> - It compared parotid-sparing IMRT (the PARSPORT trial) versus conventional radiotherapy
> - It demonstrated a reduction in grade 2–4 xerostomia scores with IMRT at 12 and 24 months (29% vs. 83% at 24 months)

Further reading

Bernier J, Cooper JS, Pajak TF, et al. Defining risk levels in locally advanced head and neck cancers: a comparative analysis of concurrent post-operative radiation plus chemotherapy trials of the EORTC (#22931) and RTOG (#9501). Head Neck 2005; 27:843–850.

Bourhis J, Overgaard J, Audry H, et al. Hyperfractionated or accelerated radiotherapy in head and neck cancer: a meta-analysis. Lancet 2006; 368:843–854.

Nutting CM, Morden JP, Harrington KJ, et al. Parotid-sparing intensity modulated versus conventional radiotherapy in head and neck cancer (PARSPORT): a phase 3 multicentre randomized controlled trial. Lancet Oncol 2011; 12:127–736.

Pignon JP, le Maître A, Maillard E, et al. Meta-analysis of chemotherapy in head and neck cancer (MACH-NC): an update on 93 randomised trials and 17,346 patients. Radiother Oncol 2009; 92:4–14.

Long case 17: Maxillectomy and DCIA flap

The patient in this figure had resective surgery 9 months ago.

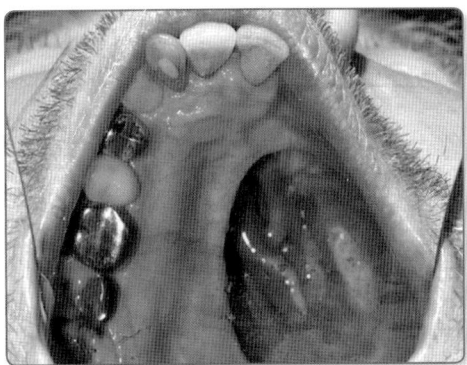

17.1 Question

How would you assess this patient?

Answer

- Correct positioning
- History
- Examination
- Review of investigations
- Management plan

17.2 Question

What are the key points in the history?

Answer

- Reason for surgery: neoplasia, non-neoplastic lesion, trauma
- Adjunctive treatment: radiotherapy, chemotherapy
- Medical history: fitness for operation
- Drug history: requiring modification of surgery chosen
- Social history: family support, smoking

17.3 Question

What are the key points in the examination?

Answer

- Resection site: structures involved
- Neck dissection scar
- Lymphadenopathy or recurrence
- Defect in hard and soft palate
- Oro nasal and oro-sinus communication
- Donor site morbidity

17.4 Question
How would you classify the defect?

Answer
- Maxillary defects classically classified according to Brown (Box A)
- A DCIA commonly used for Class 3 and 4 defects

17.5 Question
What further assessment is required?

Answer
- Assessment requirement for neck dissection: review imaging and histology (Box B)
- Speech and language assessment: swallow and speech
- Patient's wishes for treatment
- Virtual surgical planning (Box C)

17.6 Question
What are the reconstructive options?

Answer
- Soft tissue only
- Hard tissue only
- Hard +/– soft tissue: DCIA, fibula, scapula
- Obturator (Box D)
- Implants placement (Box E)

17.7 Question
You agree on a DCIA flap due to the shape of the maxillary defect. What are the advantages?

Answer
- Large volume of high-quality bone to accommodate osseointegrated implants
- Contour matching lateral mandible
- Potential for generous skin paddle
- Muscle mucosalises well intraorally

17.8 Question
What are the possible complications of a DCIA flap?

Answer
- Recipient site: sinusitis, speech and swallowing difficulty
- Donor site: sensory loss and/or neuropathy in the lateral thigh and inguinal region, hernia formation
- Implants: failure (Box E)

Box A. Brown and Shaw's classification of maxillectomy defects (2010)

- Maxillectomy not causing an oronasal fistula
- Not involving the orbit
- Involving the orbital adnexae with orbital retention
- With orbital enucleation or exenteration
- Orbitomaxillary defect
- Nasomaxillary defect
- Palatal defect only, not involving the dental alveolus
- Less than or equal to 1/2 unilateral
- Less than or equal to 1/2 bilateral or transverse anterior
- Greater than 1/2 maxillectomy
- The system can be used to guide reconstructive options, for instance the DCIA or TDAP flaps lending themselves to class IV defects in particular with muscle bulk allowing mucosalised closure of the oral fistula

Box B: Treating maxillary tumours with neck dissections

- Traditionally there has been a lower propensity to offer neck dissections in patients with maxillary tumours
- Brown et al. reported in 2013 however that incidence of nodal metastases for maxillary alveolus and hard palate was similar to elsewhere in the oral cavity (37% vs. 40%)
- Higher regional recurrence rates (26% vs. 7%) were found due to the tendency not to perform elective neck dissections in this cohort (Montes and Schmidt 2008)

Box C: Virtual surgical planning

- Virtual surgical planning with segments of the Iliac crest matched to the anticipated maxillectomy defect allow for custom cutting guides. Enables either custom-made plates or adaption of reconstruction plates using a printed model
- Preplacement of implants has been utilised prior to flap harvest or placed with a printed surgical stent: maximises aesthetics and function and reduces operating time
- Preoperative planning with CT angiography helps harvesting of perforator flaps

Box D: Obturator or DCIA?

- Maxillectomy defects may occur in patients whose general health precludes complex free flap transfer
- Obturators offer a reasonable alternative
- Breeze et al. (2016) demonstrated no significant different in health-related quality of life in 39 consecutive patients treated with free flaps or obturators
- This was similar to a previous study by Rogers et al. (2003)

> **Box E: Success rates of osseointegrated implants in the DCIA?**
> - Success rates are comparable to scapula and fibula
> - A review by Burgess et al. (2017) demonstrated 95% success overall
> - Success rates in composite flaps as a whole is variable in the literature (70–99%)

Further reading

Beahm EK, et al. Iliac flap. In: Wei F-C, Mardini S (Eds) Flaps and Reconstructive Surgery Elsevier Saunders, 2009.

Breeze J, Rennie A, Morrison A, et al. Health-related quality of life after maxillectomy: obturator rehabilitation compared with flap reconstruction. Br J Oral Maxillofac Surg 2016; 54:857–862.

Brown JS, Bekiroglu F, Shaw RJ, et al. Management of the neck and regional recurrence in squamous cell carcinoma of the maxillary alveolus and hard palate compared with other sites in the oral cavity. Head Neck 2013;35:265–269.

Thomas CV, McMillan KG, Jeynes P, et al. Use of a titanium cutting guide to assist with raising and inset of a DCIA free flap. Br J Oral Maxillofac Surg 2013; 51:958–961.

Chapter 3

Orthognathic surgery

SHORT CASES

1. Taking an orthognathic patient history
2. Examination of the orthognathic patient
3. Use of imaging in orthognathic surgery
4. Preoperative assessment and planning in orthognathic surgery
5. Inverted L osteotomy
6. Hemimandibular hyperplasia
7. Low angle class II skeletal relationship
8. High angle class III skeletal relationship
9. Postoperative sagittal split osteotomy
10. Condylar resorption following sagittal split osteotomy
11. Segmental osteotomy
12. Transverse maxillary deficiency

LONG CASE

13. High angle class II skeletal relationship

Short case 1: Taking an orthognathic patient history

A patient has been referred to your clinic for potential orthognathic surgery.

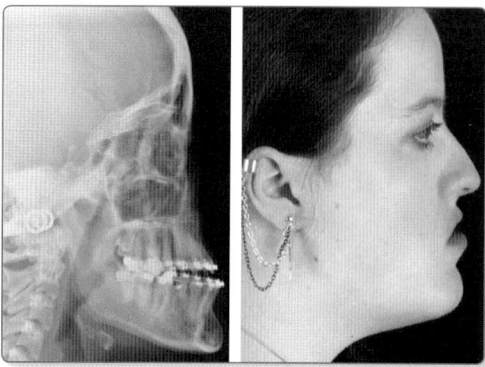

1.1 Question
What are the key points in the history?

Answer
- Referral source (Box A)
- Presenting complaint
- History of presenting complaint (Box B)
- Previous temperomandibular joint (TMJ) symptoms
- Previous orthodontic treatment
- Previous dental treatment
- Previous surgical treatment
- Past medical history
- Drug history
- Social history
- Expectations of treatment
- Summarise back to the patient

1.2 Question
How would you assess this patient further?

Answer
- Ask 'What has brought you in to see us today?'
- Type of clinician making the referral (Box A)
- Function and/or appearance (face and/or teeth)

1.3 Question

What specific TMJ symptoms should you ask about?

Answer

- Pain when chewing
- Clicking
- Previous treatment
- Trauma to TMJ

1.4 Question

What questions about any previous orthodontic treatment are relevant?

Answer

- Removable or fixed appliances
- Tooth extractions
- How long the braces was worn for
- Compliance

1.5 Question

What questions about any previous dental treatment are relevant?

Answer

- Ongoing care or past treatment
- Assessment of risk for caries or periodontal disease

1.6 Question

What questions about any previous surgical treatment are relevant?

Answer

- Third molars removed
- Prior orthognathic surgery
- Existing altered sensation to lip, chin or tongue as result of surgery

1.7 Question

What questions about the patient's past medical history are relevant?

Answer

- Comorbidities relevant to anaesthetic or surgical risk
- Allergies
- Psychiatric issues (Box C)

1.8 Question

Why are questions about their drug history relevant and how would you manage anticoagulants?

Answer

- Relevant to intra- or postoperative complications
- Anticoagulation should be discussed with a haematologist to see whether they can be potentially omitted

1.9 Question

What questions about the patient's social history are relevant?

Answer

- Support in immediate postoperative period
- Effect of surgery on relationships
- Occupation

1.10 Question

Why is it important to ascertain the patient's expectations of treatment?

Answer

- Patient must be clear on expectations
- Ensure expectations are realistic
- Clarify if evidence of secondary gain (such as improvement in a relationship or work)

Box A: Potential sources for referral

- General dental practitioner: pointed out by clinician or patient
- Orthodontist: general practice, specialist practice, secondary care
- General medical practitioner
- Other clinician: e.g. respiratory physician for obstructive sleep apnoea (OSA)

Box B: History of the presenting complaint

- Congenital or acquired
- Progression
- Chewing and eating
- Occlusion
- Previous trauma: to bones or teeth
- Childhood infections
- OSA (Box B)
- Effect on quality of Life

> **Box C: Tailored OSA history**
>
> - Assessment by respiratory physicians: this is essential before consideration of treatment
> - Symptoms: snoring, daytime sleepiness
> - Mandatory preoperative assessments: polysomnography, apnoea–hypopnoea index (AHI) and Epworth Sleepiness scale (ESS) questionnaires
> - Previous nonsurgical treatment: avoidance of alcohol, weight loss, continuous positive airway pressure (CPAP) devices, protrusive mandibular splints
> - Previous surgical treatment: uvulopalatopharyngoplasty, hyoid advancement, midline glossectomy

> **Box D: Tailored psychiatric history**
>
> - The most challenging component of an orthognathic assessment
> - Previous or current mental health problems are not a contraindication to treatment but must always be carefully explored
> - Questions must come naturally from you and should therefore be practiced
> - A simple question might be as follows 'we ask all patients coming in for this type of surgery the same question as it is important we choose the correct treatment for you. One of these questions is that I have to ask you if you have ever suffered from problems with your mental health?'

Further reading

Bailey LJ, Proffit WR, White R Jr. Assessment of patients for orthognathic surgery. Semin Orthod 1999; 5:209–222.

Short case 2: Examination of the orthognathic patient

This patient has presented to the joint orthognathic clinic following referral from their orthodontist.

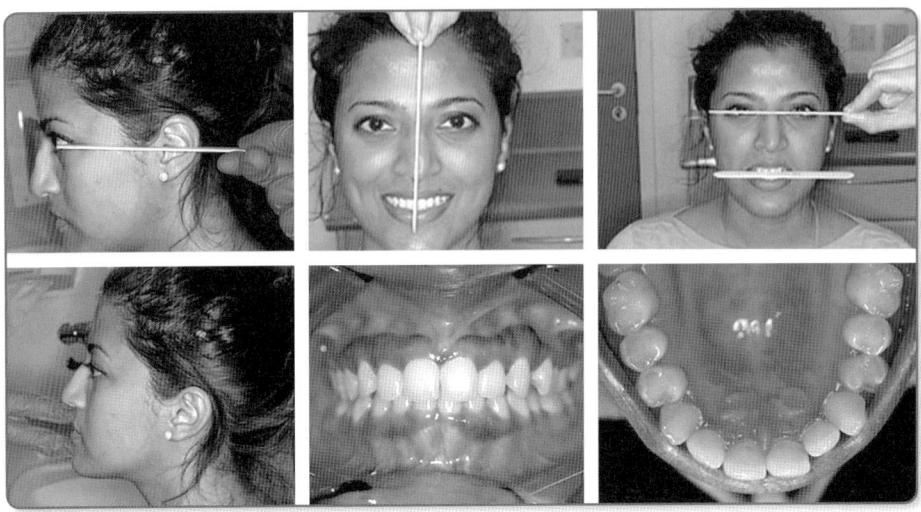

2.1 Question

What are the sequential steps of an examination for potential orthognathic surgery in a newly presenting patient as shown in the figure?

Answer

- Preparation
- Examination from the front
- Examination from the side
- Examination from behind
- Intraoral examination

2.2 Question

What steps are required in preparation?

Answer

- Patient sitting upright (Box A)
- Frankfort plane level to floor/or neutral head position
- Remove camouflage: hair over face, hats, glasses
- Confirm if a syndromic case

2.3 Question

How would you examine the patient from the front?

Answer

- Symmetry: use a spatula placed intercanthally

- Facial fifths (Box B)
- Vertical proportions (Box C)
- Maxillary cant
- Upper lip length
- Incisor show at rest
- Incisor show dynamic
- Dental centre line: should be coincident with facial midline
- Lip competence
- Lower lip to chin length
- Lower dental midline: coincident with face and/or chin
- Chin asymmetry

2.4 Question

How would you examine the patient from the side?

Answer

- Skeletal class (Box D)
- Fronto nasal angle
- Scleral show and malar projection
- Nasolabial angle
- Labiomental angle
- Chin throat length
- Chin shape

2.5 Question

How would you examine the patient from behind?

Answer

- Symmetry
- Scleral show
- TMJ palpation

2.6 Question

How would you perform the intraoral examination?

Answer

- Oral hygiene
- Overjet
- Overbite
- Upper to lower dental centre lines
- Teeth present
- Crowding
- Pathology
- Deviation on closing

2.7 Question

How would you summarise your findings?

Answer
- Summarise (Box E)
- Study models
- Radiographs
- Treatment plan

Box A: Measuring facial fifths

- Lines drawn vertically from medial and lateral canthi, lateral aspect of alar bases and canine teeth tips
- Intermedial canthal distance = alar base width = intercanine width

---

Box B: Measuring vertical proportions

- Anterior versus posterior facial heights
- Posterior facial height: utilises the Frankfort mandibular plane angle
- Anterior facial height: utilises anterior facial thirds
- Middle anterior: glabella to subnasale
- Lower anterior: subnasale to soft tissue menton
- Anterior lower facial third is further subdivided into: upper third (subnasale to stomion) and lower two-thirds (stomion to soft tissue menton)

Box C: Measuring skeletal class

- "Please put your tongue to the roof of mouth, close teeth until just about to touch"
- Skeletal class: fingers into A and B points (1, 2 or 3)

Box D: Mean examination values (Caucasian)

- Middle anterior third (45%), lower anterior third (55%)
- Upper lip length: 22 mm (males), 20 mm (females)
- Incisal show at rest: 2 mm (males), 3 mm (females)
- Lower lip to chin length: 44 mm (males), 40 mm (females)
- Overjet: 2–4 mm (class I), >2 mm (class II), <2 mm (class 3)
- Nasolabial angle: 90–110 degrees (less in males, greater in females)

Short case 2 Examination of the orthognathic patient

> **Box E: Summarising**
>
> This must be brief and not simply repeating the assessment. A suggested outline is as follows:
> - Patient complaint
> - Pertinent medical and social history
> - Syndromic or not
> - Symmetrical or not
> - Skeletal class
> - Problem lies in maxilla or mandible or both?
> - Low, normal or high angle
> - Plan
>
> For example: 'This patient dislikes how prominent her front teeth are. They are medically well and are currently at university. On examination, this is a nonsyndromic symmetrical patient with a low angle class II skeletal relationship with mandibular hypoplasia. My orthodontic plan is to align, level and coordinate. My surgical plan is to perform a bilateral sagittal split osteotomy (BSSO) to advance to a class I incisal relationship'.

Further reading

Wolford LM. Surgical Planning in Orthognathic Surgery and Outcome Stability. In: Brennan P, Schliephake H, Ghali G, Cascarini L (Eds). Maxillofacial Surgery, 3rd Edition, 2017.

Short case 3: Use of imaging in orthognathic surgery

This patient attends your clinic to discuss what plan will be undertaken for their forthcoming orthognathic surgery.

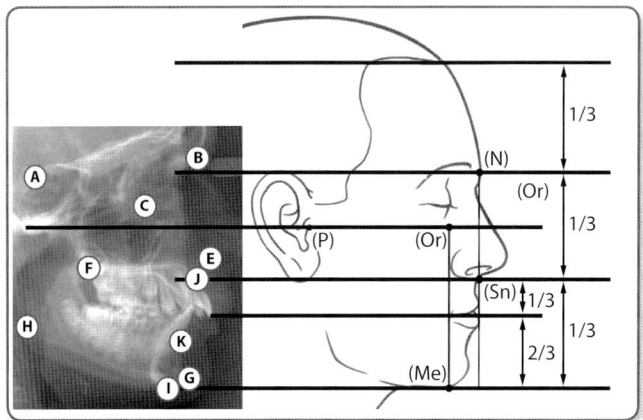

3.1 Question

What types of imaging should be requested prior to orthognathic surgery?

Answer

- Lateral cephalogram
- OPG
- Periapical radiograph
- Occlusal radiograph
- CBCT

3.2 Question

What are the practical concepts of taking a lateral cephalogram?

Answer

- Standardised and reproducible method of determining angles and measurements that can be compared to mean values for a particular population
- Ear rods placed in external auditory meatus
- Image is taken with Frankfort plane horizontal and teeth in maximum intercuspation
- Dose is 6 microsieverts (lower than OPG)

3.3 Question

Name the commonly used cephalometric points labelled in the figure?

Answer

- A: Sella: centre of sella turcica
- B: Nasion: most anterior point of fronto-nasal suture
- C: Orbitale: most inferior anterior point on margin of orbit
- D: Porion: uppermost point on bony external auditory meatus
- E: Anterior nasal spine (ANS): most anterior point (the tip) of hard palate
- F: Posterior nasal spine (PNS): most posterior point of bony hard palate
- G: Pogonion: most prominent point on contour of chin in sagittal plane
- H: Gonion: projected point on mandible of bisected angle between a line along lower mandibular border and line down posterior ramus border
- I: Menton: most inferior point on mandibular symphysis
- J: A point: position of deepest concavity on anterior profile of maxilla
- K: B point: position of deepest concavity on anterior profile of mandibular symphysis

3.4 Question

What are the commonly used lines on a lateral cephalogram?

Answer

- Cranial base: sella to nasion (SN)
- Maxillary plane: ANS to PNS
- Mandibular plane: gonion to mention
- Frankfort plane: highest point on the upper margin of the external auditory canal and the lowest point on the lower margin of the orbit
- Middle anterior facial height (nasion to ANS)
- Lower anterior facial height (LAFH, ANS to menton)

3.5 Question

What are the commonly used cephalometric measurements?

Answer

- Maxillary-mandibular plane angle (MMPA): 27 ± 5 degrees
- Frankfort-mandibular plane angle (FMPA)
- LAFH/TAFH ratio: approximately 50–55%
- SNA: 81 degrees (relationship of maxilla to cranial base)
- SNB: 79 degrees (relationship of mandible to cranial base)
- ANB: 2–4 degrees (class I), >4 degrees (class II), <2 degrees (class III)
- Upper central incisor (U1) inclination: 109 degrees
- Lower central incisor (L1) inclination: 120 degrees minus MMPA (mean of average 93)

3.6 Question

Describe simplistically how you would determine whether it is the maxilla or mandible that is positioned wrongly?

Answer

- Steiner analysis: relating the cranial base (S–N) to A and B points (SNA and SNB)

- McNamara Analysis: a line is dropped down from nasion perpendicular to Frankfort plane. The distance from this line to A point is measured (normal value is 1 mm ahead)
- Ricketts zero-meridian line: with the Frankfort plane horizontal, drop a vertical line from Nasion and relate that line to pogonion. Pogonion lies behind line in skeletal class II and in front in class III

3.7 Question

What parameters would you check on an OPG?

Answer

- Third molars: presence or absence
- Pathology: cysts, caries, bone levels and root lengths
- Position of the inferior alveolar (IA) nerve: to assist in positioning lingual surgical cut

3.8 Question

When would you request periapical radiographs?

Answer

- These should be taken if diagnosis of tooth condition is suspicious (especially suspected short roots)

3.9 Question

When would you request an occlusal radiograph?

Answer

- To assess position of unerupted canine tooth, in conjunction with OPG

3.10 Question

When would you request a cone beam CT?

Answer

- For three-dimensional (3D) virtual planning, including cutting guides
- Printing 3D models
- Bending custom plates
- Assess position of displaced teeth including canines and potential effect on adjacent teeth

3.11 Question

What is your protocol for follow-up imaging post-surgery?

Answer

- Refer to BAOS/BAOMS guidelines (Box A)

> **Box A: BAOS/BAOMS guidelines for follow-up imaging post-surgery**
> - Prior to discharge post-surgery: OPG
> - 1–3 weeks: lateral cephalogram
> - 6 months (prior to debonding): lateral cephalogram

Further reading

Bell RB. Computer planning and intraoperative navigation in cranio-maxillofacial surgery. Oral Maxillofac Surg Clin North Am 2010; 22:135–156.

Levine JP, Patel A, Saadeh PB, et al. Computer-aided design and manufacturing in craniomaxillofacial surgery: the new state of the art. J Craniofac Surg 2012; 23:288–293.

Short case 4: Preoperative assessment and planning in orthognathic surgery

The patient in the figure below is due to attend clinic tomorrow for final planning prior to orthognathic surgery.

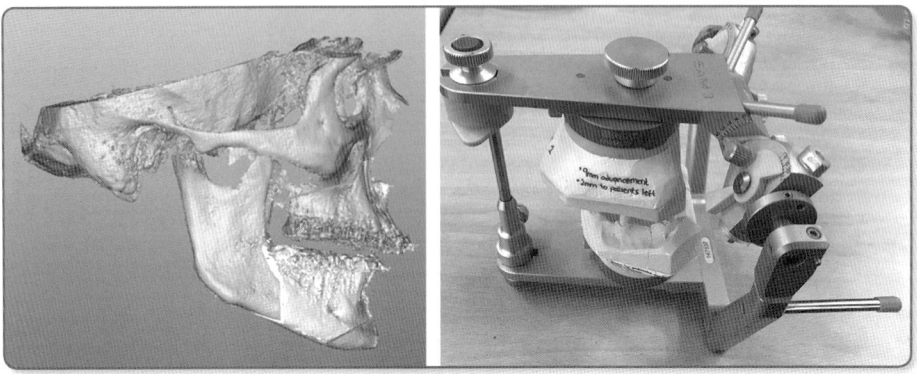

4.1 Question

The orthodontist feels the patient is ready for surgery. What surgical preparation is required?

Answer

- Impressions for articulated study models
- Inter occlusal registration (physical impression or hand-held scanner)
- Face bow
- Clinical photographs
- Imaging (case 3)
- Surgical hooks
- Consent
- Blood tests
- Letter to orthodontist
- Planning: articulator with physical models or virtual surgical planning (Box A and D)
- Specific tests for obstructive sleep apnoea (Box B)

4.2 Question

What pre-operative blood tests would you request?

Answer

- Refer to the NICE guidance 2016 (Box A)
- All patients should have full blood count and urea and electrolytes
- There is no evidence to support either a group and save, cross match or even a coagulation screen in American Society of Anaesthesiologists (ASA) grade I patients who have no history of bleeding disorders or previous blood transfusion

4.3 Question

Can you identify any common pitfalls in the assessment?

Answer

- Posturing mandible: when assessed clinically, during lateral cephalogram, or during bite registration
- Pseudo mandibular prognathism in low angle class III patient that overcloses: patient should be reassessed with mouth open slightly so chin less pronounced
- Occlusal cant
- Incorrect measurements using facebow

4.4 Question

What is your overall rationale for planning of soft and hard tissue movements?

Answer

- Orthognathic surgery moves bones of facial skeleton (Box C)
- Aesthetic result is determined by soft tissue profile
- Both hard and soft tissue movements must be planned and anticipated

4.5 Question

Using the articulator shown in the figure, how would you sequentially plan the required movements?

Answer

- Movements usually planned as they will be performed surgically (Box D)
- Move maxilla if not positioned correctly; otherwise no maxillary surgery required
- Check mandible in right place once maxilla is moved
- Check chin in right place once mandible is moved
- Assess resultant effects on overlying soft tissues

4.6 Question

Using the articulator how would you plan your maxillary bony movements?

Answer

- Anteroposterior: move upper incisor tip to ideal position – advancement will increase incisor show
- Vertical (anterior): determine position of upper incisor tip, defined by degree of vertical maxillary excess and upper incisor show at rest (beware of short upper lip)
- Vertical (posterior): impaction to close anterior open bite (AOB)
- Vertical (lateral): presence of cant will necessitate impaction or downward positioning of one side more than other
- Transverse: maxillary expansion may be required
- Rotational (horizontal plane): used to correct upper dental centreline discrepancies

4.7 Question
Using the articulator how would you plan the mandibular bony movements?

Answer
- Anteroposterior: move mandible to class I incisal relationship (consider edge-to-edge incisors if large movement and orthodontist requests some 'planned' relapse)
- Vertical and anteroposterior: based upon autorotation to new maxilla position
- Transverse: assess lower dental centreline in relation to upper dental centreline and facial midline

4.8 Question
Using the articulator how would you plan the chin bony movements?

Answer 4.8
- Anteroposterior: recognise that posterior movements often have poor aesthetic results
- Vertical: effect on facial height

4.9 Question
What are the predicted nasal changes with maxillary surgery?

Answer
- Width: broadened (impaction)
- Nasal tip: upturned (advancement)

4.10 Question
How does the nasal tip move relative to the A point?

Answer
- 1:3 for osteotomies at the LeFort I level
- 1:2 for osteotomies at the LeFort II level
- 1:1 osteotomies at the LeFort III level

4.11 Question
What upper lip movements would you predict in a standard LeFort I level osteotomy?

Answer
- Advancement: 80% of skeletal move
- Setback: 50% of skeletal move
- Impaction: 10–40% of bony impaction
- Affected by lip morphology, e.g. thick lip moving less than thin lip
- Scarred lip (e.g. cleft) may move in ratio of 1:1

4.12 Question

Where would you predict the lower lip position to be following mandibular osteotomy?

Answer

- Affected by many factors and difficult to predict
- Does not follow lower incisor teeth in predictable pattern
- Estimates of ~85% of skeletal move in advancement and 60% in set-back quoted

4.13 Question

What are the predicted chin soft tissue movements following osteotomy, genioplasty or alloplastic implant?

Answer

- BSSO: soft tissue pogonion to bone pogonion moves consistently in a 1:1 fashion with either BSSO advancement or setback
- Advancement genioplasty: 100% (i.e. 1:1)
- Alloplastic augmentation: soft tissue moves 80–90%

Box A: Virtual surgical planning

- Two-dimensional (2D) planning utilises a lateral cephalogram and clinical photographs
- Three-dimensional planning utilises a CT or CBCT, and often 3D surface photography
- Three-dimensional planning will likely replace conventional surgical planning eventually
- The occlusion is imported by scanning casts (less accurate) or direct intraoral scanning
- It is cheaper per patient after initial set up costs
- It is likely to be more accurate for complex cases: asymmetry and maxillary cant
- Splints, surgical cutting guides and prebent plates can be made for the maxilla
- If a CBCT is used then radiation doses are similar to plain radiographs

---

Box B: Orthognathic surgery to treat OSA

- Advancement of the mandible and/or maxilla and/or genioplasty
- Results in anteroposterior and lateral expansion of airway
- Degree of necessary advancement is debated (>10 mm suggested)

Box C: Broad surgical options

- Mandible: BSSO, VSS, Segmental, Inverted L, Genioplasty
- Maxilla: LeFort (1, 2, 3), Kufner, Segmental

> **Box D: Articulators**
> - Types of articulator commonly used include: simple, semi adjustable, fully adjustable
> - Adjustable articulators are recommended in particular for bimaxillary surgery, and those cases with a maxillary cant
> - Specific articulators (such as the SAM 3) are made for orthognathic surgery
> - The facebow reading is a key component in accurate model surgery

Further reading

Garg M, Coleman M, Dhariwal DK. Are blood investigations, or group and save, required before orthognathic surgery? Br J Oral Maxillofac Surg 2012; 50:611–613.

National Institute for Health and Care Excellence. Routine preoperative tests for elective surgery [NG45]. London 2016.

Verbraecken J, Hedner J, Penzel T. Pre-operative screening for obstructive sleep apnoea. Eur Respir Rev 2017; 143:26.

Short case 5: Inverted L osteotomy

This patient has returned for follow-up 6 weeks postoperatively

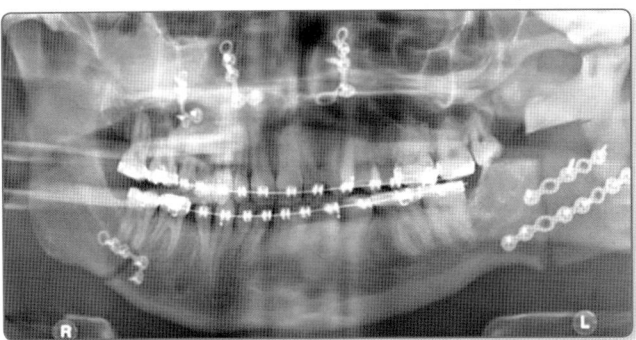

5.1 **Question**

What are your observations from the radiograph of this patient shown in the above figure?

Answer

- OPG radiograph demonstrating a patient post-orthognathic surgery
- Maxillary osteotomy at LeFort 1 level with three L-shaped plates
- BSSO on right side
- Inverted L osteotomy on left side

5.2 **Question**

What are the postoperative key points?

Answer

- Preoperative concerns
- Type of surgery performed: cutaneous incision, semi rigid plates or intermaxillary fixation
- Complications from surgery: numbness, facial weakness

5.3 **Question**

How would you examine this postoperative patient?

Answer

- Assess patient from front, side and above
- Skeletal class: aiming for class I
- Anterior facial height is unchanged
- Facial symmetry: preoperative deviation of chin to left corrected
- Check maxillary cant corrected by procedure
- Scar: from external approach

- Facial nerve weakness: from external approach
- Occlusion
- Donor bone graft site: likely iliac crest

5.4 Question
What are the indications for an inverted L osteotomy?

Answer
- Decreased posterior face height requiring posterior vertical changes
- Large mandibular movements
- Large asymmetry
- Abnormal ramus anatomy, e.g. syndromic patients
- 'Bird-face' deformities can be treated by this procedure as they lack posterior facial height (Box A–C)

5.5 Question
What are the advantages of an inverted L osteotomy, as opposed to a conventional BSSO?

Answer
- Able to lengthen the posterior face height
- Reduced risk to IA nerve (6% permanent risk each side)

5.6 Question
What are the disadvantages of an inverted L osteotomy?

Answer
- Requirement for bone grafts in most cases: usually from the iliac crest
- External approach: scar, risk to facial nerve
- Requirement for IMF for 6 weeks if not plated

5.7 Question
What are the key points in the procedure?

Answer
- Both intraoral or extraoral approaches are used (Boxes D and E)
- Bone grafts are usually required and taken from the iliac crest
- Patients can be plated or placed in IMF

Box A: Features of a 'bird face' deformity
- Significant class II skeletal base
- Increased FMPA
- Marked mandibular retrogenia
- Reduced posterior face height
- Radiologically diminutive condyles

Box B: Challenges with treating a 'bird face' deformity with a conventional BSSO
- Large mandibular advancement often required: stability, technically difficult to plate
- This may increase an already high anterior facial height
- High propensity for relapse: high angle, large movements, abnormal condyles

Box C: Treatment options for a 'bird face' deformity traditionally include
- Conventional BSSO
- Inverted 'L' osteotomy
- Distraction osteogenesis

Box D: Concept of an extraoral approach
- Upper Risdon or retromandibular incision
- Greater access for cuts with standard drill or saw
- Template used to guide position of cuts
- Easier positioning and fixation of bone grafts
- Fixation of fragments with miniplates or prebent heavier profile plate

Box E: Concept of an intraoral approach
- Standard BSSO incision
- Endoscopic visualisation
- Right angled drill
- Insertion of bone graft
- IMF or semi rigid fixation with plates
- Fixation using right angled screwdriver or transbuccal trocar with stab incision

Further reading
Barer P, Wallen T, McNeill R, Reitzik M. Stability of mandibular advancement osteotomy using rigid internal fixation. Am J Orthod Dentofacial Orthop 1987; 92:403–411.

Greaney L, Bhamrah G, Sneddon K, Collyer J. Reinventing the wheel: a modern perspective on the bilateral inverted 'L' osteotomy. Int J Oral Maxillofac Surg 2015; 44:1325–1329.

Short case 6: Hemimandibular hyperplasia

This patient has been referred by their dentist for assessment of their facial asymmetry.

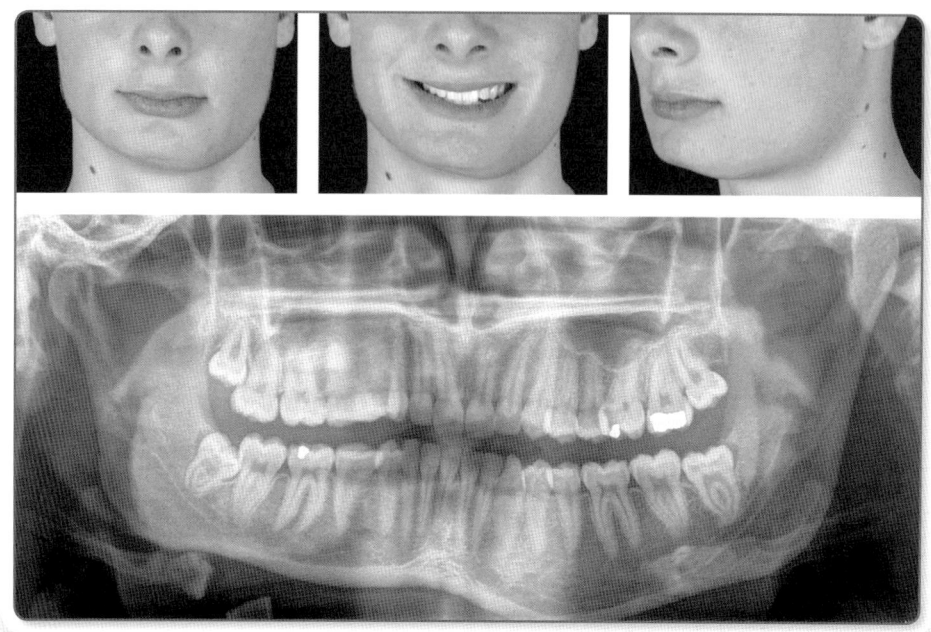

6.1 Question

What are the key points in assessing this patient who dislikes the asymmetry of his face?

Answer

- Patient has mandibular asymmetry; causes are diverse (Box A)
- Orthographic assessment required by taking a tailored history, examination and review of pertinent investigations
- Need to differentiate between hemimandibular elongation (HE) and hemimandibular hyperplasia (HH)

6.2 Question

What are the key points in the history?

Answer

- Duration of problem: developmental, pathological, traumatic (Box A)
- Ongoing changes: facial asymmetry, occlusal changes
- Previous treatment: surgical, orthodontic
- TMJ symptoms: HH often causes TMJ pain and contralateral joint clicking

6.3 Question

What are the key points in the examination?

Answer

- Assess patient from front, side and above
- Skeletal relationship: class I relationship suggestive of HH
- Facial height: likely anterior vertical proportions
- Maxillary cant: present and therefore suggestive of HH
- Midlines: upper and lower dental centre lines and chin centre point are all coincident with facial midline

6.4 Question

What investigations would you request to confirm the nature of the disease and determine progression?

Answer

- Serial study models
- Serial height measurements
- Cervical Maturation Index
- Imaging: OPG, CT, SPECT
- Photographs: clinical and patient's own
- Laser facial surface scanning

6.5 Question

Can you comment on the appearance of this OPG of the patient?

Answer

- Condylar head size: increased size on left (expected in HH)
- Condylar neck length: no difference
- Ramus height: increased height suggestive of HH (measure from mesial cusp of first molar tooth to the lower border straight through the root on each side)
- IA nerve position: no clear difference (would expect to be inferiorly positioned in HH)

6.6 Question

What is the role of CT in differentiating HH from HE?

Answer

- CT will demonstrate an increase in size of one half of mandible in three dimensions in HH
- It will also identify pathological lesions

6.7 Question

What is SPECT and what is its role in assessment of mandibular asymmetry?

Answer

- SPECT uses intravenous technicium radio-isotope
- Aims to distinguish normal bone turnover within condyle from increased activity that may be cause of asymmetry
- A relative percentage uptake of 55% or more in affected mandibular condyle considered abnormal

6.8 Question

What are the treatment options for this 16-year-old male patient?

Answer

- Treatment options are shown in Box B
- Interceptive treatment: far more indications with HH than HE
- Camoflague (if mild) or surgery (once sure not progressing)
- Maxillary surgery: differential transverse impaction to correct cant
- Mandibular surgery: asymmetrical BSSO and/or genioplasty

Box A: Causes of mandibular asymmetry

Developmental
- Hemimandibular elongation
- Hemimandibular hyperplasia
- Condylar hyperplasia
- Hemifacial microsomia
- Hemifacial hypertrophy
- Torticollis
- Dental crossbite causing deviation of mandible

Pathological
- Tumours: osteochrondroma
- Cysts
- Fibro-osseous lesions
- Infection
- Condylar resorption
- Hemifacial atrophy (Parry–Romberg syndrome)

Traumatic
- Condylar fractures

Box B: Differences between HE and HH

Table 1

Variable	Hemimandibular hypertrophy (HH)	Hemimandibular elongation (HE)
Condylar head	Increased size – causes TMJ pain and contralateral joint clicking	Normal
Condylar neck	Increased size	Increased length
Ramus	Increased height	Normal
Body	Increased height	Longer ipsilaterally
IA nerve	Inferiorly positioned	Normal
Skeletal class	Usually 1	Usually 3
Maxilla	Grows downwards resulting in a cant but still in occlusion unless rapid mandibular growth	May get late canting as result of cross/scissor bite
Chin point and dental midline	Apparent deviation to ipsilateral side	True deviation to contralateral side
Open bite	Usually lateral if rapid growth	No
Occlusion	Normally class I but with vertical discrepancies, e.g. canting + lateral open bite	Ipsilateral scissor bite and contralateral cross bite
Treatment	Interceptive: high condylar shave, functional appliance Orthodontic camouflage: if mild Orthognathic surgery	Interceptive: high condylar shave Orthodontic camouflage Orthognathic surgery

Further reading

Hodder SC, Rees JI, Oliver TB, Facey PE, Sugar AW. SPECT bone scintigraphy in the diagnosis and management of mandibular condylar hyperplasia. Br J Oral Maxillofac Surg 2000; 38:87–93.

Obwegeser HL, Makek MS. Hemimandibular hyperplasia- hemimandibular elongation. J Maxillofac Surg 1986; 14:183–208.

Posnick JC, Perez J, Chavda A. Hemimandibular Elongation: Is the Corrected Occlusion Maintained Long-Term? Does the Mandible Continue to Grow? J Oral Maxillofac Surg 2017; 75:371–398.

Short case 7: Low angle class II skeletal relationship

This patient is being seen in joint orthognathic clinic shortly prior to orthognathic surgery.

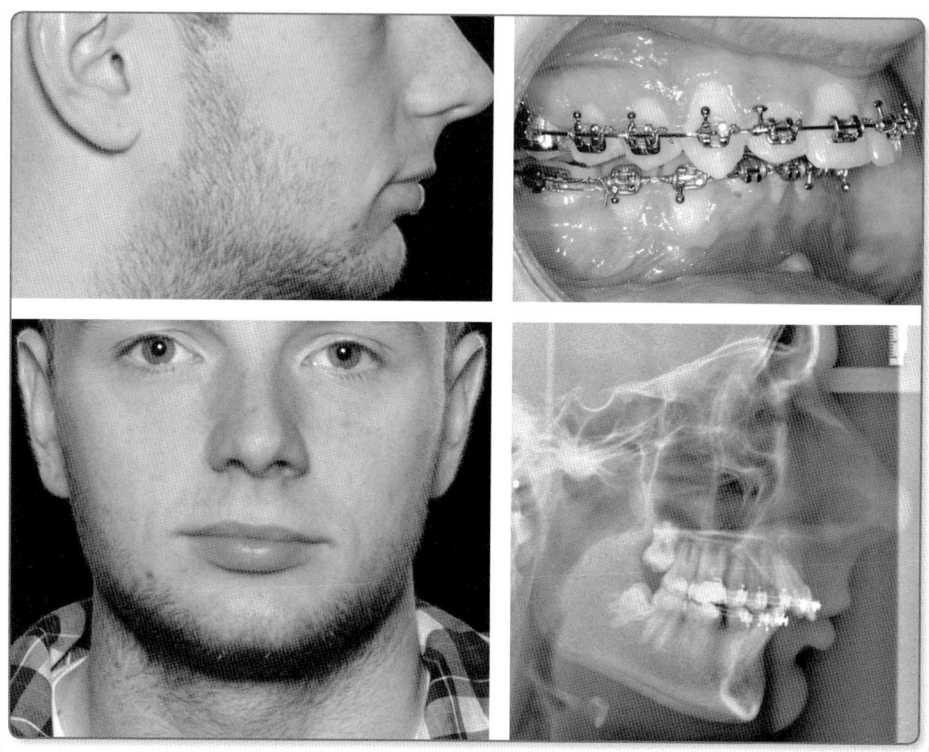

7.1 Question

What are the key points in examining this patient?

Answer
- Assess patient from front, side and above (Box A and B)
- Class II division II incisal relationship
- Class II skeletal relationship
- Decreased FMP angle
- Decreased LAFH
- Lip trap and increased labiomental fold
- Lip incompetence at rest with mentalis hyperactivity

7.2 Question
How could you confirm a low angle without formally measuring it?

Answer
- In normal angle, lines should intersect at the occiput; in low angle, lines will intersect more posteriorly

7.3 Question
What cephalometric features can you see?

Answer
- Decreased LAFH
- Decreased MMPA
- Normal SNA
- Decreased SNB
- Increased ANB

7.4 Question
How would you treat a low angle class II patient due to a retrognathic mandible?

Answer
- Treatment options are orthodontics alone or surgery plus orthodontics (Box C)
- Assess and discuss patient in MDT setting and agree on orthodontic and surgical objectives

7.5 Question
What pre-surgical orthodontics would you expect the patient to have had?

Answer
- Decompensate: incisor angulations (turn into class II division I relationship)
- Alignment
- Coordination: of arches
- Relief of crowding: possible need for extraction of mandibular premolars
- Some clinicians extract mandibular third molars in preparation for osteotomy

7.6 Question
What is the importance in decompensating the incisors in this case?

Answer
- Increasing overjet enables a larger surgical movement
- Addresses the underlying skeletal relationship

7.7 Question

What are the surgical objectives?

Answer

- BSSO advancement to a class I incisal relationship (Box D)
- Aim for a three-point landing to increase LAFH
- A reduction and downwards genioplasty may be required additionally

7.8 Question

Based on an 11-mm overjet, how much would you advance the mandible?

Answer

- Aim to produce a class I incisal relationship with overjet of approximately 2–3 mm
- This approximates to a 10-mm movement
- Some clinicians set the wafer to an edge-to-edge relationship, recognising there may be some intraoperative 'sagging' of condyles

7.9 Question

What is the expected soft tissue movement with this surgery?

Answer

- In both an advancement and setback BSSO, the soft tissue pogonion to bone pogonion moves consistently in a 1:1 fashion

---

Box A: Concept of a class II skeletal relationship

- Caused by either a retrognathic mandible (low angle) or vertical maxillary excess (high angle)
- The major aetiological factor is genetic
- There is a small environmental component: allergy, respiratory function, atypical swallowing, chronic mouth breathing, thumb sucking behaviour

---

Box B: Common features in a low angle class II skeletal relationship

- Class II incisal relationship
- Incisors either division I (proclined) or division II (retroclined)
- Class II skeletal relationship
- Normal or decreased FMP angle
- Normal or decreased LAFH
- Lip trap and increased labiomental fold
- Lip incompetence at rest with mentalis hyperactivity
- Decreased chin throat length
- Increased or traumatic overbite
- Crowded lower labial segment with fan shaped incisors

> **Box C: Treatment options for a low angle class II skeletal relationship**
>
> During growth
> - Growth modification: functional appliance (e.g. twin block), 'low pull' headgear
>
> Growth complete
> - Orthodontic camouflage: extraction (usually upper premolars) or nonextraction (mild discrepancies)
> - Mandibular osteotomy
> - Bimaxillary osteotomy with clockwise rotation to soften chin point

> **Box D: Surgical options for a low angle class II skeletal relationship**
> - BSSO
> - Inverted 'L' ramus osteotomy
> - Distraction

Further reading

Proffit WR. Treatment of skeletal problems in children. In: Proffit WR: Contemporary orthodontics, 4th Edition Elsevier 2007.

Tulloch J, Phillips C, Proffit WR. Benefit of early Class II treatment: Progress report of a two-phase randomized clinical trial. Am J Orthod Dentofacial Orthop 1998; 113:62–72.

Short case 8: High angle class III skeletal relationship

The patient shown in the figure who dislikes his chin and is being assessed for a potential osteotomy.

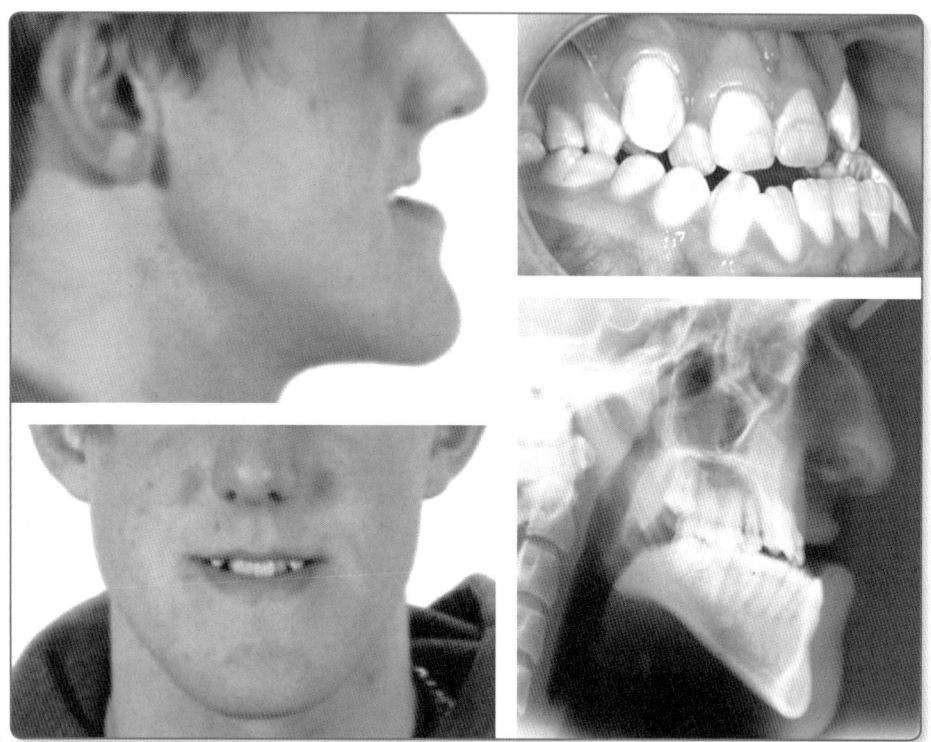

8.1 **Question**

What are the key points in examining this patient? Do not focus on the history and assume the patient is fit and well.

Answer

- Examination comprises extra (Box A), intraoral (Box B) examination, followed by a summary (Box C)

8.2 **Question**

What would be your proposed treatment plan?

Answer

- Bimaxillary osteotomy
- Maxillary advancement and anterior maxillary impaction
- Setback of mandible to a class I incisal relationship

8.3 Question
Can you estimate how much movement the maxilla will likely require?

Answer
- Straight AP movement of mandible would be 3 mm alone
- With autorotation this will likely necessitate a 4–5 mm movement
- Anterior maxillary impaction of 2 mm required to produce an incisal show at rest of approximately 2 mm
- Physical or virtual model surgery required to predict such movements

8.4 Question
What are some potential consequences of these movements?

Answer
- Impaction and advancement of maxilla may upturn nasal tip and widen nose respectively
- Autorotation may result in an over projected chin, necessitating genioplasty

8.5 Question
When would you perform genioplasty?

Answer
- Some clinicians suggest performing at same time and others suggest waiting. Review the patient at six months (Box D)
- Treatment at same time prevents requirement for second surgery but is more difficult to predict movement, and numbness reportedly higher

8.6 Question
Is it possible to treat the patient with just single jaw surgery?

Answer
- Maxilla is hypoplastic in AP dimension and requires advancement
- 7 mm maxillary advancement alone would over project the maxilla
- 7 mm mandibular setback would not address hypoplastic maxilla and would result in poor aesthetics in terms of chin throat length

Box A: Key extraoral features in this case

- Symmetrical
- High angle (increased facial height)
- Skeletal class III
- Reduced nasolabial angle
- No obvious maxillary cant
- Normal upper lip length of 22 mm
- Incisor show at rest of 3 mm
- Upper dental centre line is coincident with facial midline
- Lips are incompetent at rest
- Increased lower lip to chin length
- No chin asymmetry

Box B: Key intraoral features in this case

- Reverse overjet of 5 mm
- Normal overbite
- Good oral hygiene with no obvious dental caries or periodontal disease
- Upper to lower dental centrelines
- Teeth present except the third molars
- Crowding in the maxillary anterior segments
- Lower dental midline coincident with face and chin

Box C: A suggested summary of this case

- This is a nonsyndromic symmetrical high angle class III patient with a hypoplastic maxilla and a 4-mm reverse overjet

Box D: Follow-up of patients post osteotomy

- Patients should be followed by a surgeon for 6 months
- No recommendations currently exist to recommend the frequency
- In the absence of complications a commonly utilised regime is: 1 week, 2 weeks, 4 weeks, 6 months
- The BOS/BAOMS imaging protocol is recommended (see chapter 4.3)

Further reading

Huang CS, Hsu SS, Chen YR. Systematic review of the surgery-first approach in orthognathic surgery. Biomed J 2014; 37:184–190.

Short case 9: Postoperative sagittal split osteotomy

This patient had surgical correction of a class II skeletal relationship with anterior open bite 4 weeks ago?

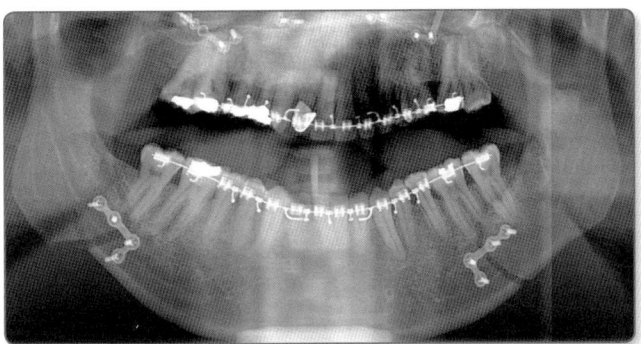

9.1 Question
Please comment on the radiograph of this patient.

Answer
- OPG radiograph of patient following BSSO and LeFort 1 osteotomy
- Bilateral L shaped Plates with two screws on either side of fracture line
- A step on he lower border on right side
- Third molar teeth extracted prior to the osteotomy as sockets have healed
- Unable to comment on occlusion
- Inadequate radiograph as unable to see condyles

9.2 Question
Is there any further information you would want to know?

Answer
- History: planned surgical movement
- Examination: malocclusion, complications post-surgery (Box A)
- Additional OPG to see if condyles are in fossa

9.3 Question
The patient had an asymmetrical BSSO, both condyles are in the fossa and the occlusion is good. How would you comment on the step in the right body?

Answer
- If correcting a cant, right distal segment may have been repositioned superiorly which could have resulted in a step in lower border

9.4 Question

Do you remove third molars before an osteotomy?

Answer

- No evidence that removal of third molars prior to BSSO affects incidence of bad splits
- Many clinicians still remove third molars approximately 6 months before osteotomy

9.5 Question

Where do bad splits occur and how are they managed?

Answer

- Most common bad split occurs when buccal cortex breaks off (up to 5%) but only problematic in advancements where bony overlap of buccal segment with distal fragment required
- Unfavourable splits to lingual cortex generally prevent use of interpositional screws
- Coronoid splits require no treatment
- Condylar neck splits are rare and require condyleotomy and either plating of condyle to correct fragment or more commonly a period of IMF followed by repeat surgery if planned movements cannot be achieved

9.6 Question

What can you do to ensure favourable splits?

Answer

- Ensure bony cuts are through mandibular cortex in all areas
- Ensure complete cut of lower border cortex with drill, saw or piezoelectric device (Box C)
- Careful propagation of split with chisels and spreaders

9.7 Question

How would you quantify the risks of permanent damage to the IA nerves?

Answer

- Percentages are per nerve
- Temporary alteration of sensation is very common: from 50–80%
- Long-term complete absence sensation (analgesia): 10%
- Long-term reduced touch appreciation (hypothesia): 20%
- Troubling altered sensation (paraesthesia and dysaesthesia) may occur
- Increased risks listed in Box B

Box A: Potential complications post BSSO

- Generic: pain, infection, bleeding, swelling
- Inferior alveolar nerve damage
- Lingual nerve damage
- Rarely facial nerve damage: more common with mandibular setback
- Bad split and need for IMF
- TMJ dysfunction (see Scenario 4.10)
- Malocclusion
- Relapse (see Scenario 4.10)
- Trismus

Box B: Risk factors for increased risk of IA nerve numbness

- Additional genioplasty
- Inferior alveolar nerve closer to buccal cortex on CT scan
- Increasing age of patient
- Use of chisels on the lingual cortex
- Bicortical screws
- May be reduced incidence with use of piezo saw

Box C: Modifications of BSSO

- Trauner and Obwegeser (1957): introduced the concept of BSSO, with horizontal lingual and buccal cuts
- Dal Pont (1961): changed buccal cut from horizontal to vertical
- Hunsuck (1968): shorter lingual cut reduces chance of the distal fragment impinging in the pterygomasseteric sling in large set-backs
- Epker (1977): complete osteotomy of the lower border reduces the chance of a bad split

Further reading

Bruckmoser E, Bulla M, Alacamlioglu Y, et al. Factors influencing neurosensory disturbance after bilateral sagittal split osteotomy: retrospective analysis after 6 and 12 months. Oral Surg Oral Med Oral Pathol Oral Radiol 2013; 115:473–482.

Doucet J, Morrison AD, Davis BR, et al. The presence of mandibular third molars during sagittal split osteotomies does not increase the risk of complications. J Oral Maxillofac Surg 2012; 70:1935–1943.

Ow A, Cheung LK. Bilateral sagittal split osteotomies versus mandibular distraction osteogenesis: a prospective clinical trial comparing IA nerve function and complications. Int J Oral Maxillofac Surg 2010; 39:756–760.

Short case 10: Condylar resorption following sagittal split osteotomy

The patient shown in the figure is 1-year post-osteotomy and is complaining that her chin is becoming less prominent and the gap between her teeth is getting bigger again.

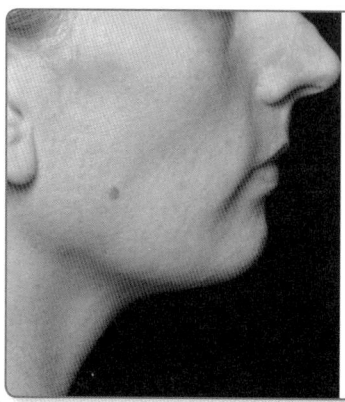
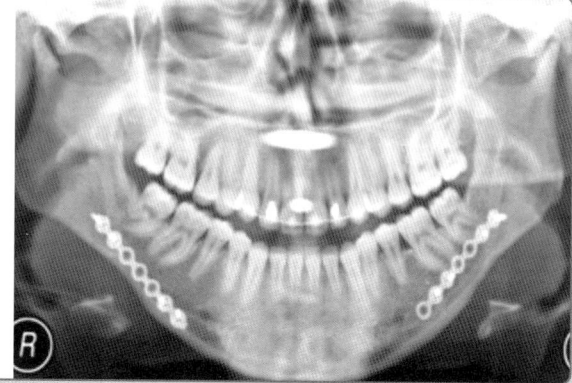

10.1 Question

The patient shown in the figure is 1-year post-osteotomy and is complaining that her chin is becoming less prominent and the gap between her teeth is getting bigger again. How would you assess them?

Answer

- Potential causes include failure of fixation (early), relapse or migration (late)
- Assessment involves focused history, examination and review of imaging

10.2 Question

What are the key points in the history?

Answer

- Type of procedures performed: single jaw, bimaxillary, type of movement
- Time postprocedure: days or months
- When problem first noticed: early or late
- Complications of surgery: numbness, altered occlusion, infection
- Presurgical TMJ symptoms

10.3 Question

The patient had a BSSO a year ago. What are the key points in the examination?

Answer

- Extraoral
- Skeletal class: class II
- FMP angle

- Lip and tongue numbness
- LAFH
- Intraoral: occlusion; evidence of infection or plate exposure

10.4 Question

What is likely to have happened and what are the risks?

Answer

- Patient has had late relapse (Box B)
- Expect increased overjet and possible decrease in lower posterior face height
- Approximately 5% of BSSO advancement osteotomies >7 mm get a degree of relapse
- Early relapse occurs within 6–8 weeks and is attributed to movement at osteotomy site
- Late relapse occurs between 6 and 17 months and often attributed to condylar resorption

10.5 Question

What observations can you make from this recent radiograph?

Answer

- Bilateral plate fixation
- Likely post BSSO and the osteotomy sites have healed
- Small and flattened condylar heads
- Clinical presentation consistent with bilateral condylar resorption

10.6 Question

What are the risk factors for idiopathic condylar resorption following BSSO?

Answer

- Incidences for idiopathic condylar resorption are very varied (1–31%)
- See Box B

10.7 Question

What other factors apart from condylar resorption affect the risk of relapse?

Answer

- Mandibular advancement more stable than setback (Box C and D)
- Larger advancements less stable (>7 mm) than smaller movements
- Previous surgery increases risk of relapse

10.8 Question

How do you manage idiopathic condylar resorption?

Answer

- Wait for it to 'burn out' as it is believed to be hormonally driven

- Monitor with serial radiographs and study models
- Soft diet
- Retrusive jaw exercises
- Lower bite raising appliance to disclude joint from function
- Steroids
- Request a SPECT scan once burned out to check for bone turnover
- Once patient has stabilised consider further surgery, but again risk of relapse
- Some clinicians suggest joint replacement is better option

Box A: Key definitions

Stability
- Maintenance of the achieved postoperative result in the long term
- Post-surgical change may be classified as relapse or migration

Migration
- Continued movement in the direction of the initial move

Relapse
- Movement towards the preoperative position
- May be skeletal or dental in origin
- Pre-surgical orthodontics aims to build in relapse

Box B: Risks for condylar resorption following mandibular osteotomy

- Large advancements (reportedly >10 mm)
- Class II skeletal relationship
- Female sex
- High MMPA
- Previous TMJ dysfunction
- Counter clockwise rotation of the condyles

Box C: Factors affecting relapse following maxillofacial osteotomy

- Direction of movement: hierarchy of stability (Box D)
- Size of movement: >7 mm advancement in either the maxilla is mandible is less stable.
- Previous surgery
- Cleft
- Condylar resorption: higher in females
- Fixation methods: fixed better than wires (no difference between screws and plates)
- Period of IMF: may help

> **Box D: Proffit's hierarchy of stability (most stable first)**
> - Maxillary impaction
> - Mandibular advance
> - Maxillary advancement
> - Maxillary impaction with mandibular advancement
> - Maxillary advancement with mandibular set-back
> - Mandibular set-back
> - Maxillary transverse increase width
> - Inferior positioning of maxilla

Further reading

Ow A, Cheung LK. Skeletal stability and complications of bilateral sagittal split osteotomies and mandibular distraction osteogenesis: an evidence-based review. J Oral Maxillofac Surg 2009; 67:2344–2353.

Posnick JC, Fantuzzo JJ. Idiopathic condylar resorption: current clinical perspectives. J Oral Maxillofac Surg 2007; 65:1617–1623.

Proffit WR, Turvey TA, Phillips C. The hierarchy of stability and predictability in orthognathic surgery with rigid fixation: an update and extension. Head Face Med 2007; 3:21.

Short case 11: Segmental osteotomy

This patient returns to clinic for final review prior to planned surgery next week.

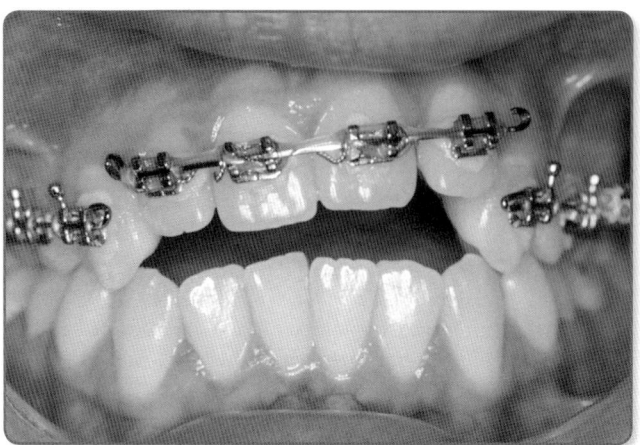

11.1 Question

What surgery does the patient shown in the figure probably have planned for next week?

Answer

- Archwire on incisal teeth sectioned at junction with canines
- Segmental maxillary osteotomy

11.2 Question

Do you think the patient is ready for surgery next week?

Answer

- Possibly too early for surgery as there is no archwire on lower arch and the lower arch is not yet leveled and aligned
- Also there is no space between crowns of laterals and canines and root torquing of teeth to create room for saw cuts

11.3 Question

What other orthodontic preparation is required for such cases?

Answer

- Level, align, coordinate and decompensate each individual segment separately (Box A)
- Create space for cuts or plan extraction of teeth during surgery

11.4 Question

What are the advantages of a maxillary segmental osteotomy?

Answer

- Facilitates correction of very localized occlusal defects
- Provide a single stage correction of transverse defects, without requirement for surgically assisted rapid palatal expansion (SARPE) followed by separate LeFort 1 osteotomy

11.5 Question

What are the potential complications of a whole or segmental maxillary osteotomy?

Answer

- Exessive bleeding
- Tooth damage (more common in segmental)
- Avascular necrosis (more common in segmental)
- Numbness: cheek skin and teeth (3% permanent)
- Nasal changes (Box B)
- Lip changes: flattening or increased prominence
- Base of skull complications: e.g. cranial nerve palsy including blindness
- Altered speech: large movements and clefts
- Relapse
- Malunion: usually inferior movements

11.6 Question

What methods do you know to lessen widening of the nasal base?

Answer

- Alar cinch suture (Box C)
- Alar sill reduction/contouring
- Sub spinal osteotomy: keep nasal musculature attached to bone by detaching anterior nasal spine (ANS) from body of maxilla, removing the need to strip bone off ANS

11.7 Question

How will impacting the anterior maxilla affect the upper lip?

Answer

- Lip length will reduce 10–40% of bony impaction (Box D)

11.8 Question

What movements cause upturning of the nasal tip and how can it be reduced?

Answer
- The nasal tip may upturn with an advancement
- Trimming the anterior nasal spine may prevent upturning (Box B)

Box A: Components of pre-surgical orthodontics

- Relieve crowding: extractions, expansion, interproximal reduction
- Levelling of occlusal plane: may not alter if changing lower face height in a three point landing
- Align arches
- Elimination of tooth rotations
- Decompensation of incisors
- Coordinate arches: so teeth will interlock post-surgery
- Build in relapse

Box B: Potential nasal changes with maxillary movements

- Alar base: widens with impaction
- Nasal tip: upturns with advancement
- Deviation: septum may buckle with impaction
- Nasolabial angle: decreases with maxillary advance
- Nasal length: may appear to increase with maxillary advancement

---

Box C: Predicted movement of the nasal tip relative to A point

- 1 to 3: at LeFort I level
- 1 to 2: at the Le Fort II level
- 1 to 1: at the Le Fort III level

Box D: Predicted movements of the upper lip for LeFort I level osteotomy

- Advancement: 80% of skeletal move
- Setback: 50% of the skeletal move
- Impaction: 10–40% lip shortening
- Downward: lip lengthens by approximately 50%
- Affected by lip morphology, e.g. thick lip moving less than thin lip
- Scarred lip (e.g. cleft) may move in a ratio of 1 to 1

> **Box E: Relapse**
> - Impaction is the most stable movement
> - Stability decreases if combined with advancement
> - Larger moves are less stable (particularly >8 mm)
> - A period of IMF may aid stability
> - Inferior positioning has relapse rates of 30–50%
> - Bone grafting may enhance stability in inferior repositioning

Further reading

Arpornmaeklong P, Heggie A. A comparison of the stability of single-piece and segmental LeFort I maxillary advancements. J Craniofac Surg 2003; 14:3–9.

Ho MW, Boyle MA, Cooper JC, et al. Surgical complications of segmental LeFort I osteotomy. Br J Oral Maxillofac Surg 2011; 49:562–566.

Short case 12: Transverse maxillary deficiency

The patient shown in the figure dislikes the appearance of his upper teeth.

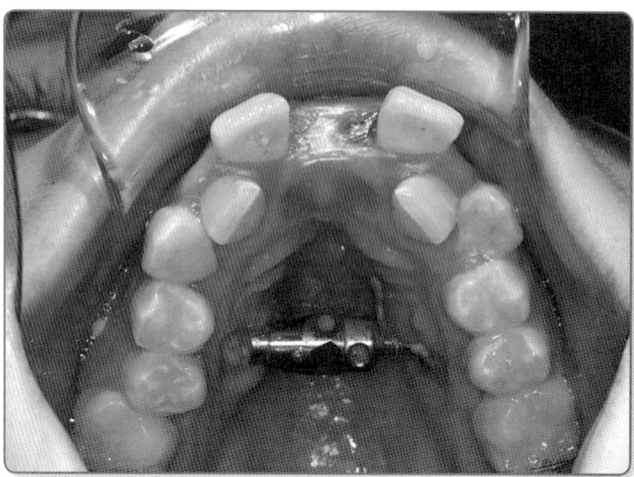

12.1 Question

What are the key points of assessment in the above patient?

Answer

- This patient has a bone anchored device, used for widening the maxilla
- They have probably had a SARPE

12.2 Question

How would you assess this patient?

Answer

- Tailored history, examination and review of investigations

12.3 Question

What are the key points in the history?

Answer

- Presenting complaint: crowded teeth, potentially difficulty in biting, unhappy with appearance of teeth/face
- Previous orthodontic treatment: this procedure is usually performed prior to fixed appliances
- Previous surgical treatment: extraction of teeth
- SARPE surgery: time post-surgery, complications, patient compliance with turning of appliance

- Past medical and drug history
- Social history, including compliance

12.4 Question

What are the key points in the examination?

Answer

- Assess patient from front, side and above
- Determine skeletal relationship, facial height, interarch width discrepancy, crowding
- Surgical complications post SARPE: condition of periodontium around upper incisors, stability of appliance, infection, numbness, teeth damage or mobility

12.5 Question

What investigations would you like to review?

Answer

- Study models: estimate arch discrepancy and thereby amount of distraction required
- Imaging: trace lateral cephalogram to aid planning, whether further surgery is required or if can be corrected by orthodontics alone

12.6 Question

What other options for expansion are there?

Answer

- Orthodontically or surgically (Box A and B)
- Corresponds to the degree of expansion required, i.e. an arch wire can perform small movements only; and the age of the patient (palatal suture closes in teenage years)

12.7 Question

What are the broad concepts of the SARPE?

Answer

- Standard LeFort I horizontal cuts but no down fracture
- Apply distractor and open until tense (Box C and D)
- Perform midline vertical cut the length of palate
- Open distractor until incisors start to move and then release by 2 mm
- Latent period: 2–3 days
- Activation: patient rotates appliance screw twice daily (each a 0.5 mm movement)
- End point is when maxillary palatal cusps sit in intercuspal groove of mandibular molar teeth
- Expansion is often over-corrected by 2 mm to account for relapse
- Compensation: appliance is left in situ for 10–12 weeks

Box A: Options for management of transverse arch discrepancy
- Orthodontic expansion: arch wire alone (mild), quad helix (moderate), rapid maxillary expansion (severe)
- Surgical expansion: segmental osteotomy, SARPE

Box B: Indications for treatment
- Patients in whom the mid-palatal suture has fused (at around 14 years of age) and who are thus not suitable for rapid palatal expansion by orthodontic means alone
- Large movements: up to 15 mm movement possible

Box C: Advantages of each type of surgical distractor
- Tooth borne device: quicker surgical time
- Bone borne: less buccal tipping, better patient comfort (as smaller), can commence orthodontics whilst device is still in situ

Box D: Advantages of a segmental over SARPE
- Single stage correction of maxilla hypoplastic in both AP and transverse dimensions: prevents requirement for additional LeFort 1 osteotomy
- Correction of AOB caused by posterior maxillary excess
- Need for differential movement of segments of maxillary dentition

Box E: Indications for maxillary distraction
- Anterior: congenital cases with significant maxillary hypoplasia, e.g. Crouzons, Aperts, Pfeifers, hemifacial microsomia, cleft lip and palate
- Anterior: obstructive sleep apnoea: brings soft palate forwards
- Inferior: post-traumatic
- Widening: SARPE

Further reading
Chamberland S, Proffit W. Closer look at the stability of surgically assisted rapid palatal expansion. J Oral Maxillofac Surg 2008; 66:1895–1900.

Long case 13: High angle class II skeletal relationship

The patient shown in the figure has been referred for orthognathic surgery.

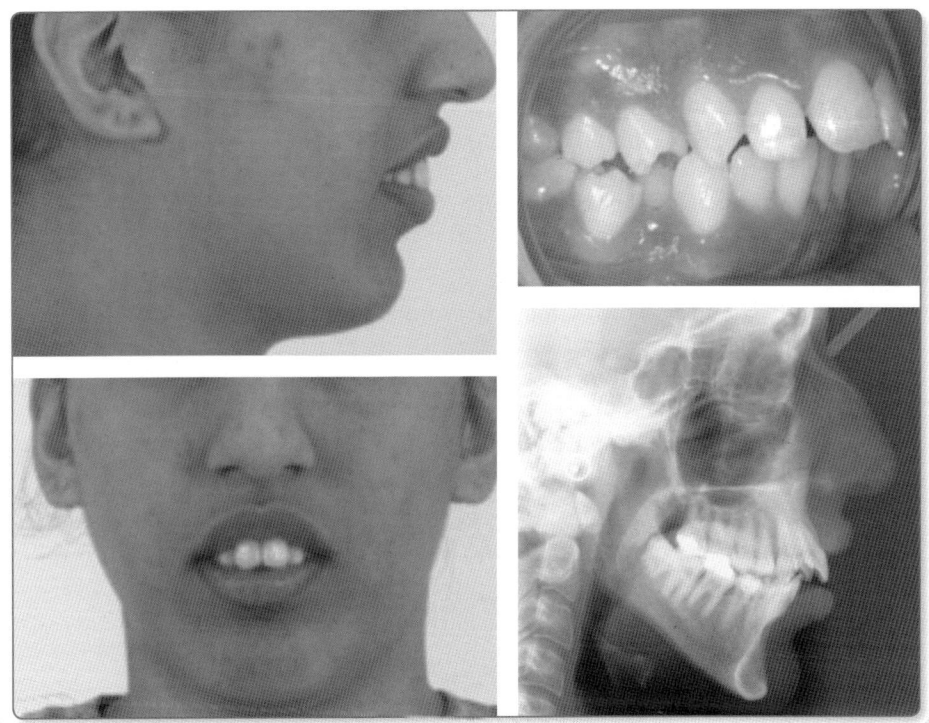

13.1 Scenario (Box A)
Please assess them and provide your proposed management plan?

13.2 Preparation
- Use time to introduce yourself, clean your hands and obtain consent to assess
- Position patient and try to come to a spot diagnosis

13.3 History
- Slow yourself down, build rapport, try not to miss key points such as social history
- Do not be tempted to rush straight into examination

13.4 Examination
- Assess from front, above, side and below (Box B)
- Use provided ruler to measure distances
- Do not be afraid to write findings down

- Do not forget to mention oral hygiene and dental health
- Key findings in a high angle class II relationship are shown in Box B

13.5 Investigations

- If articulator present ensure you pick it up and comment on it
- If investigation missing ask for it
- Articulated study models
- Plain films: OPG, lateral cephalogram
- Photographs: progression
- Three-dimensional printed model

13.6 Treatment

- Thank patient and turn directly to examiner and summarise your findings
- Orthodontic objectives (Box C)
- Surgical objectives (Box D)
- Emphasise need for multidisciplinary management
- Potential topics for discussion include postoperative stability and aetiology of condition

---

Box A: Concept of the orthognathic long case

- A 15-minute assessment likely encompassing the structure above
- The patient will inevitably be pre-surgery, but may have started orthodontics or surgical maxillary expansion
- An orthognathic scenario is highly likely for one of the two long cases

---

Box B: Commonly seen clinical features in a high angle class II skeletal relationship

- Class II skeletal base but can be class III
- High FMPA
- AOB or tendency towards one if edge to edge
- Increased LAFH
- Narrow (often 'V' shaped) maxillary arch
- Crowded upper labial segment
- Full arch crossbite
- Increased incisal show
- Hypoplastic maxilla in AP direction causes dorsal nasal hump due to retropositioned ANS
- Class II incisal relationship
- Incompetent lips
- Buccal corridors

> **Box C: Orthodontic objectives**
>
> - Relieve crowding: extraction of upper premolars (usually take out 5s but take 4s if more space required)
> - Decompensation: correct incisor angulation
> - Coordination of arches: may need arch expansion
> - Alignment

> **Box D: Surgical objectives**
>
> - Impact maxilla: differential posterior if no VME, impact all maxilla if VME
> - Advance maxilla slightly: allows fragments to override and thereby making impaction easier
> - Autorotate mandible
> - Potentially set back or advancement of mandible depending on degree of autorotation

Further reading

Solano-Hernández B, Antonarakis GS, Scolozzi P, Kiliaridis S. Combined Orthodontic and Orthognathic Surgical Treatment for the Correction of Skeletal Anterior Open-Bite Malocclusion. JOMS 2013; 71:98–109.

Chapter 4

Facial cutaneous surgery

SHORT CASES

1. Cutaneous malignancy history
2. Examination of a facial skin lesion
3. Eyelid reconstruction
4. Melanoma
5. Nasal reconstruction
6. Temple reconstruction
7. Scalp reconstruction following squamous cell carcinoma

LONG CASE

8. Auricular reconstruction

Short case 1: Cutaneous malignancy history

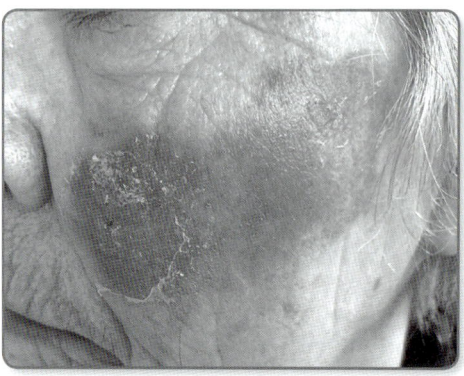

1.1 Question
What are the key features when taking a history from a patient presenting with a potentially malignant facial cutaneous lesion?

Answer
- Establish history of the lesion, whether it has appeared de novo or within pre-existing mole
- If changes to a pre-existing mole, characterise what these were (e.g. size, shape, bleeding, itchiness, etc.)
- Ask about childhood history of sunburn (notable risk factor for melanoma)
- Lifelong sun exposure including occupation (think about compensation for certain occupations, e.g. military) and sunbed use
- Previous treatment: types (surgery, radiotherapy, chemotherapy, immunotherapy) and complications to date and any related issues
- Drug history: including vitamin D supplements (Box A)
- Familial history: melanoma, dysplastic nevus syndrome (Box B), pancreatic cancer

1.2 Question
Which patients are at an increased risk of melanoma?

Answer
- Atypical mole phenotype
- Previous melanoma
- Organ transplant recipients (or any other patient on immunosuppressants)
- Patients with giant congenital pigmented naevi
- Family history of three or more cases of melanoma or pancreatic cancer

1.3 Question
What follow-up protocol is recommended for melanoma patients?

Answer
- Limited evidence base regarding follow-up protocols for melanoma
- Patients with stage IA are seen up to 12 months at 2–4 months intervals
- All other patients should be seen 3-monthly for 3 years, then 6-monthly to 5 years
- Patients with stage IIIB and above should be seen additionally on annual basis for 10 years

1.4 Question
What is the significance of patients that are on immunotherapy drugs?

Answer
- Immune-mediated adverse reactions in immunotherapy include rash, diarrhea, vitiligo, hypopituitarism and adrenal insufficiency
- PD-1 inhibitors (e.g. nivolumab) tend to be less toxic than ipilimumab (an anti-CTLA-4)
- Ipilimumab causes colitis in 10% of recipients
- BRAF inhibitors (e.g. vemurafenib) can cause arthralgia, fatigue, diarrhoea, alopecia and secondary skin cancers (e.g. cutaneous squamous cell carcinoma in 19–26% cases)

1.5 Question
What follow-up should be offered for patients with nonmelanoma skin cancer?

Answer
- Patients with first basal cell carcinomas (BCCs) have increased risk of developing a second skin cancer (Box C)
- Patient can be discharged into community following one recall appointment
- Sun protection advice and counselling on self-examination

Box A: Vitamin D and melanoma
- All patients with melanoma should have vitamin D levels checked and supplemented if suboptimal
- Higher levels of vitamin D have been associated with lower melanoma-related mortality
- However, the nature of the relationship is uncertain, with trials ongoing in Italy and Australia

> **Box B: Dysplastic naevus syndrome**
>
> - Dysplastic naevi occur in 2–8% of Caucasian patients
> - Lifetime risk of transformation in a dysplastic naevus to malignant melanoma is estimated to be around 1/10,000
> - When restricting this to moderately-to-severely dysplastic naevi, 4% may harbor melanoma-in situ upon excision
> - In familial melanoma/dysplastic naevus syndrome, several members of the same family will present with dysplastic naevia and/or a previous history of melanoma
> - The risk for developing melanoma approaches 100% over the course of a lifetime for those family members affected
> - Complete skin examination at regular intervals and patient education in melanoma detection and prevention is recommended

> **Box C: Follow-up for nonmelanoma skin cancer**
>
> - Following a first BCC, the 3-year cumulative risk of developing a second BCC ranges from 33% to 70% (mean 44%)
> - This is a 10-fold increase over the general population
> - With regards to cutaneous squamous cell carcinoma (SCC), 75% of recurrences and metastases occur within 2 years and 95% within 5 years
> - Follow-up protocols are variable but should ideally enable monitoring of high risk tumours over this period

Further reading

Knackstedt T, Knackstedt RW, Couto R, Gastman B. Malignant melanoma: diagnostic and management update. Plast Reconstr Surg 2018; 142:202e–216e.

Marsden JR, Newton-Bishop JA, Burrows L. Revised UK guidelines for the management of melanoma 2010. Br J Dermatol 2010; 163:238–256.

National Institute for Health and Care Excellence. Melanoma: assessment and management. London: NICE, 2015.

Reddy KK, Farber MJ, Bhawan J, et al. Atypical (dysplastic) nevi: outcomes of surgical excision and association with melanoma. JAMA Dermatol 2013; 149:928–934.

Telfer NR, Knackstedt RW, Couto R, Gastman B. Guidelines for the management of basal cell carcinoma. Br J Dermatol 2008; 159:35–48.

Short case 2: Examination of a facial skin lesion

This patient has been referred for management of this lesion on their lower eyelid.

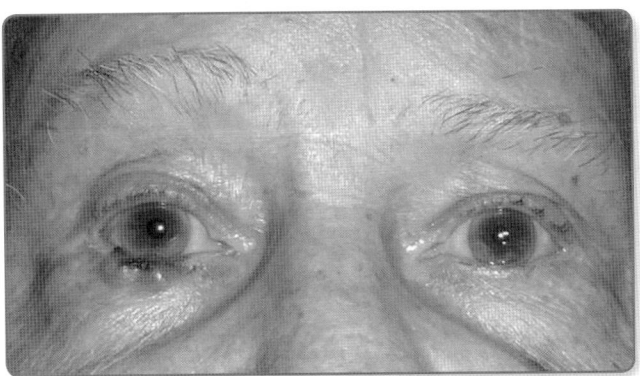

2.1 Question

What are the key features when examining a patient with a skin lesion as demonstrated in the figure?

Answer

- Pigmented versus nonpigmented
- Skin type
- Differential diagnosis
- Examine regional lymph nodes (if applicable) and parotid gland
- Dermoscopy (Box A)

2.2 Question

How are skin types classified?

Answer

- Using the Fitzpatrick classification (Box B) can help stratify risk of developing skin cancer in sun exposed individuals

2.3 Question

What diagnostic algorithms exist for differentiating melanoma from benign naevi clinically?

Answer

- ABCD rule
- Menzies method: 92% sensitivity rate for diagnosis of melanoma
- Glasgow criteria (7-point checklist)
- 3-point checklist
- CASH: colour, architecture, symmetry and homogeneity

2.4 Question

Can you describe the Glasgow criteria?

Answer

- A 7-point checklist (7PCL)
- Comprises major and minor criteria for predicting likelihood of melanoma
- Major criteria (score 2 points): changes in size, irregular border and irregular pigmentation
- Minor criteria (score 1 point): diameter 7 mm or more, inflammation, oozing/crusting, and/or change in sensation
- Score of 3 or above prompts referral

2.5 Question

How are melanomas staged?

Answer

- Using the TNM format in the AJCC 8th edition system
- T: staged by Breslow thickness and absence/presence of ulceration
- N: staged by number of nodes, whether clinically palpable or occult (i.e. sentinel node) and presence/absence of in-transit, satellite or microsatellite metastases
- M: staged by distant metastases location
- Stage IB or above should be dealt with by an SSMDT and ideally offered sentinel node biopsy

2.6 Question

Which lesions can you expect to see?

Answer

- Aim to be familiar with appearance and diagnosis of BCC, SCC, melanoma, lentigo and lentigo maligna, keratoacanthoma, Bowen's disease, actinic keratosis, Merkel cell carcinoma (rare), seborrheic keratosis and vascular anomalies
- Be familiar with alternative treatment options including radiotherapy, topical immunotherapy and chemotherapy (e.g. Efudix), curettage and cautery, cryotherapy and photodynamic therapy (PDT)

2.7 Question

What is the concept behind dermoscopy?

Answer

- Dermoscopy examines lesions more closely to achieve a more accurate diagnosis
- Lesions can be differentiated as melanocytic or nonmelanocytic

- A meta-analysis by Kittler et al. (2002) demonstrated that dermoscopy increased diagnostic accuracy for melanoma by 49%, but was significantly dependent upon skill and experience of the examiner
- A number of features are associated with increased risk of developing melanoma (Box B)

Box A: Features suggestive of increased risk of melanoma on dermoscopy

- Atypical network
- Streaks (pseudopods/radial streaming)
- Negative pigment network
- Shiny-white lines
- Atypical dots/globules
- Off-centre blotches
- Regression structures, depigmentation
- Blue-white veils
- Atypical vessels, e.g. serpentine vessels, corkscrew vessels

---

Box B: Fitzpatrick skin types

- Developed in 1975 by Thomas B. Fitzpatrick
- I: always burns, never tans (pale white skin)
- II: always burns, tans minimally (white skin)
- III: burns moderately, tans uniformly (light brown skin)
- IV: burns minimally, always tans well (moderate brown skin)
- V: rarely burns, tans profusely (dark brown skin)
- VI: never burns (deeply pigmented dark brown-black skin)

Further reading

Carrera C, Marchetti MA, Dusza SW, et al. Validity and reliability of dermoscopic criteria used to differentiate nevi from melanoma: a web-based international dermoscopy society survey. JAMA Dermatol 2016; 152:798–806.

Kittler H, Pehamberger H, Wolff K, Binder M. Diagnostic accuracy of dermoscopy. Lancet Oncol 2002; 3:159–165.

Mackie RM. Clinical recognition of early invasive malignant melanoma. BMJ 1990; 301:1005–1006.

Menzies SW, Ingvar C, Crotty KA, et al. Frequency and morphologic characteristics of invasive melanomas lacking specific surface microscopic features. Arch Dermatol 1996; 132:1178–1182.

Short case 3: Eyelid reconstruction

This is an intra-operative image of a patient you saw in clinic a week prior to surgery.

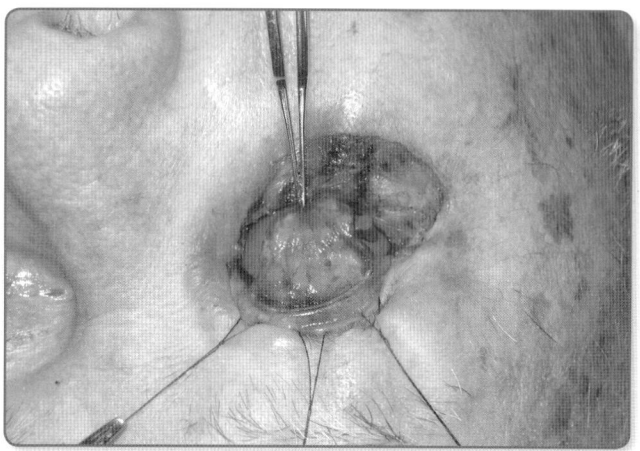

3.1 Question

What are the key features when examining a patient such as that shown in the figure?

Answer

- Lesion characteristics
- Size
- Depth: anterior or posterior lamellae
- Examination of parotid/neck as appropriate
- Differential diagnosis

3.2 Question

How will you determine appropriate treatment?

Answer

- Determine likely radial margin and depth: determines reconstructive options
- Mohs surgery: almost mandatory in this area

3.3 Question

What are the reconstructive options for upper eyelid defects?

Answer

- Smaller defects (25–30% width); direct closure in layers with key sutures repairing tarsal plate and everting margin (Box C)
- In older patients lid laxity permits direct closure in defects up to 40%

- Moderate defects (<50% width): Tenzel semicircular rotation flap, horizontal tarsoconjunctival transposition flap
- Large defects (up to 100% width): Mustarde lid switch, Cutler-Beard reserved

3.4 Question

What are the reconstructive options for lower eyelid defects?

Answer

- Smaller defects: wedge excision and primary closure (Box B)
- Moderate defects (<50% width): lateral canthotomy and cantholysis (Box A), Tenzel flap, free tarsoconjunctival graft with myocutaneous advancement where posterior lamella required
- Large defects (up to 100% width): Hughes procedure (Box D)

3.5 Question

What are the contra-indications to a Hughes procedure?

Answer

- Necessitates a period of occlusion of the visual axis
- Amblyopia-prone patients and monocular vision are contraindications to procedure

3.6 Question

What are the potential complications of upper eyelid repairs post-Mohs?

Answer

- Eyelid notching
- Ptosis
- Dehiscence
- Rounded lateral eyelid contour (failure to fix to lateral canthal ligament/ periosteal flap)
- Marginal entropion
- Eyelid retraction
- Corneal abrasion

3.7 Question

What are the potential complications of lower eyelid repairs?

Answer

- Eyelid notching
- Eyelid laxity and/or ectropion
- Conjunctival hypertrophy of the eyelid margin
- Entropion

Box A: Upper eyelid anatomy

- Both upper and lower eyelids are made up of anterior lamellae (skin and orbicularis oculi) and posterior lamellae (tarsal plate and conjunctiva)
- Deep to the orbicularis is the retro-orbicularis oculi fat (ROOF) in the upper eyelid, then the septum
- Behind the septum is the postseptal (preaponeurotic) fat pads (lacrimal gland laterally), then the levator palpebrae superioris (LPS) and aponeurosis
- Muller's muscle lies deep to this, inserting on the tarsal plate
- The levator muscle thickens behind the septum to form Whitnall's ligament

Box B: Lower eyelid anatomy

- Behind the orbicularis oculi and in front of the septum is the ROOF equivalent, the sub-orbicularis oculi fat (SOOF)
- This is followed by septum and post-septal fat as in the upper lid
- The counterpart of the LPS in the lower lid is the capsulopalpebral fascia, and Whitnall's ligament is replaced by Lockwood's
- The lower lid retractors are seen deep as fascial extensions of the inferior rectus
- Their plication providing the basis of the Jones entropion correction

Box C: Descriptions of common procedures

- Canthopexy: sutures placed to tighten a stabilise the lateral canthal tendon and orbicularis oculi, tightening the lower lid
- Canthoplasty: formal division of the lateral canthal tendon and shortening
- Cantholysis: division of the (usually inferior limb) lateral canthal tendon
- Canthotomy: division of the skin at the lateral canthal angle

Box D: The Hughes procedure

- The Hughes procedure represents an elegant solution for the full thickness defect of the lower lid
- A conjunctival flap is 'turned down' from the upper lid to replace the posterior lamella
- This is braced anteriorly by a skin graft from either the contralateral upper lid or the inner arm
- Division of the conjunctival flap is required at a second stage

Further reading

Dutton JJ. Lateral Tarsorrhaphy. In: Dutton JJ (Ed). Atlas of Oculoplastic and Orbital Surgery. Philadelphia, PA: Wolters Kluwer/Lippincott Williams & Wilkins, Health 2013: 106–107.

Hughes WL. Total lower lid reconstruction: technical details. Trans Am Ophthalmol Soc 1976; 74:321–329.

Tenzel RR, Steward WB. Eyelid reconstruction by semicircular flap technique. Ophthalmology 1978; 85:1164–1169.

Short case 4: Melanoma

This patient has been referred to you by their general practitioner.

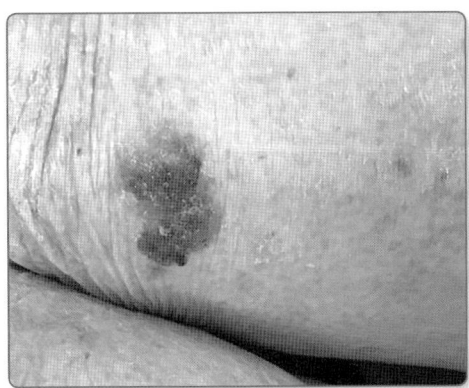

4.1 Question
What are the key features when examining the patient shown in the figure?

Answer

- Characterise subtype clinically
- Relevant nodal basins: include parotid nodes and level V nodes
- Site and size of lesion and feasibility of excision for pathology and primary closure in first instance
- Margins, pigmentation, ulceration

4.2 Question
Who should treat melanoma?

Answer

- Refer to British Association of Dermatologists (BAD) guidelines
- Criteria exist for referral from a local skin cancer MDT (LSMDT) to a specialist MDT (SSMDT)
- Criteria include patients with stage IIB disease or higher (IB if SLNB available within the network), mucosal disease, children/young adults and cases of metastatic melanoma among others

4.3 Question
What is a lentigo?

Answer

- Benign patch of pigmentation from melanocyte hyperplasia
- Distinguish from lentigo maligna (LM), which is melanoma in situ and lentigo maligna melanoma (LMM), where vertical growth and invasion have occurred

4.4 Question

How do you determine the excision margin?

Answer

- Determined by Breslow thickness (Box A)
- For a 1-cm margin for ≤1.0 mm thickness, 1–2 cm for 1.01–2.0 mm, 2–3 cm for 2.01–4.0 mm and 3 cm for anything >4 mm in thickness
- Micrographic control may be used in certain areas
- Johnson's square technique can be used for LM and LMM

4.5 Question

How should you stage and treat the neck?

Answer

- Cross-sectional imaging is not performed routinely: reserved for stage IIIB disease or higher, which should prompt CT head/chest/abdomen/pelvis
- Ultrasound-guided FNAC should be performed in first instance of suspicious nodes, although sensitivity variable (4.7–80%)
- Sentinel lymph node biopsy is recommended for stage IB and above (see Boxes B–D)
- Cervical nodal recurrence mandates modified radical neck dissection and/or extension to include (therapeutic) parotidectomy and/or posterior occipital chain where appropriate
- External jugular vein (EJV) should be excised during surgery as this is a route for distant spread

4.6 Question

What are targeted therapies and immunotherapy?

Answer

- Drugs showing significant promise in stage IV disease
- Immune checkpoint inhibitors include anti-CTLA4 (e.g. Ipilimumab) and anti-PD1 (e.g. Nivolumab) agents
- Targeted drugs include BRAF inhibitors (e.g. Vemurafenib) and MEK inhibitors

---

Box A: Melanoma prognostic indicators

- Tumour thickness (Breslow)
- Mitotic rate
- Absence/presence of ulceration
- Nodal status and tumour burden
- Presence/absence of distant metastases and location
- These are combined with age, lesion site and sex in a prediction tool accessible at www.melanomaprognosis.org)

Box B: MSLT-I

- The MSLT-I trial commenced in 1994
- It examined whether sentinel lymph node biopsy (SLNB) could be used to identify occult nodal metastases
- It compared completion lymph node dissection (CLND) following SLNB with watchful waiting and therapeutic neck dissection (TND)
- SLNB confers excellent prognostic information
- Proponents argue that SLNB strategy is associated with increased melanoma-specific survival (MSS) in node positive intermediate thickness disease, but this is contentious

Box C: Rotterdam and Dewar criteria

- Micrometastases in lymph nodes previously had a lower threshold of 0.2 mm but immunohistochemistry has changed this
- With metastases smaller than 0.1 mm now detectable, the Dewar and Rotterdam criteria were developed to characterise tumour burden by location in the lymph node (Dewar) or size of deposit (Rotterdam)
- Combining the criteria has value in predicting from a positive sentinel node the MSS and the likelihood of nonsentinel node (NSN) positivity on CLND

Box D: MSLT-II

- Examined the role of CLND in SLNB positive disease
- It increased regional disease control but did not translate to improved MSS

Further reading

Faries MB, Thompson JF, Cochran AJ, et al. Completion dissection or observation for sentinel-node metastasis in melanoma. N Engl J Med 2017; 376:2211–2222.

Morton DL, Thompson JF, Cochran AJ, et al. Final trial report of sentinel-node biopsy versus nodal observation in melanoma. N Engl J Med 2014; 370:599–609.

Newlands C, Gurney B. Management of regional metastatic disease in head and neck cutaneous malignancy. 2. Cutaneous malignant melanoma. Br J Oral Maxillofac Surg 2014; 52:301–307.

Short case 5: Nasal reconstruction

This patient presents to your clinic for suture removal at a week post surgery.

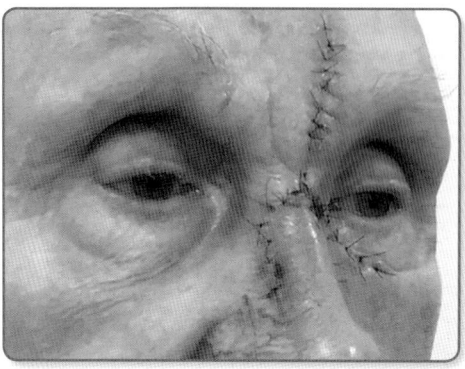

5.1 Question
What are the key features when examining the patient shown in the figure?

Answer
- Differential diagnosis of lesions and likely margin (planning the defect)
- Consideration of Mohs surgery
- Whether or not defect crosses into different nasal subunits (Box A)
- Establish whether nasal lining reconstruction and cartilage going to be required
- Examination of parotid and cervical nodes where appropriate

5.2 Question
What are the reconstructive options for nasal defects?

Answer
- Allowing defects to heal by secondary intention
- Skin grafts
- Nasolabial flap
- Bilobed flap
- Paramedian forehead flap
- Prosthetic replacement and/or osseointegrated implants (Box B)

5.3 Question
Name some potential sources of autogenous cartilage?

Answer
- Conchal bowl
- Nasal septum
- Costochondral graft

5.4 Question

What is the blood supply of the paramedian forehead flap?

Answer

- Supratrochlear artery passes under corrugator muscle at root of flap
- It becomes more superficial (subdermal) at midforehead
- Allows for flap to be thinned in this region at first stage

5.5 Question

What are the ways to minimise distortion when using a paramedian forehead flap?

Answer

- Ensure arc of rotation is as short as possible
- Restrict pedicle width to 1.5 cm
- Graft undersurface of flap at first stage to minimise contraction
- Ensure nasal lining adequately replaced (Box C)

5.6 Question

How many stages are required for a paramedian forehead flap?

Answer

- Two-stage procedure but best limited to small defects
- Debulking may be incomplete and bleeding subdermal surface prone to fibrosis and contraction
- For larger, more complex defects a three stage technique recommended
- Full-thickness, multilaminar flap is raised and primary cartilage grafts only used if vascularized nasal lining available
- Flap is physiologically delayed allowing for cartilage grafts, thinning of flap and three-dimensional sculpting of recipient bed
- Pedicle transection and final inset

Box A: The subunit approach to nasal reconstruction

- Achieving a naturalistic contour is essential
- A subunit approach to thinking about reconstruction is key
- The nose is divided into nine topographic subunits: paired sidewalls, ala and soft triangles, along with the dorsum, tip and columella
- The rule of thumb is that if a defect encompasses more than 50% of a subunit, consideration should be given to sacrificing the entire subunit in the interests of placing scars favourably and avoiding 'pin-cushioning'

Box B: Implant-retained prostheses

- Prosthetic replacements for complete rhinectomy defects may have considerable cosmetic advantages
- This is provided that patients can tolerate a removable prosthesis
- These often represent particularly good solutions when there is a more complex defect (e.g. nasomaxillary defect)
- It can be used in conjunction with composite free tissue transfer to support implants such as a composite radial, fibula
- Conventional osseointegrated implants may be placed, usually with a central implant at the radix and two further implants at the piriform region bilaterally
- Magnet or clip retainers may be used (the former are easier to locate for frailer patients, the latter arguably provide better retention)
- Zygomatic implants have been used by some, who claim excellent retention and durability

Box C: Nasal lining options

- Composite skin graft
- Advancement of residual lining
- Prefabricated forehead flap
- Folded forehead flap (modified Menick)
- A second flap, e.g. FAMM flap
- Skin graft
- Hingeover flap
- Intranasal lining flap
- Free flap: reserved for rhinectomy defects

Further reading

Menick FJ. A new modified method for nasal lining: The Menick Technique for folded lining. J Surg Oncol 2006; 94:509–514.

Menick FJ. Nasal reconstruction: Forehead flap. Plast Reconstr Surg 2004; 113:100e–111e.

Menick FJ. Nasal Reconstruction: Art and Practice, 1st Edition. Saunders, Amsterdam 2008.

Short case 6: Temple reconstruction

This patient has been referred by the dermatology team for an opinion regarding treatment of this periocular lesions.

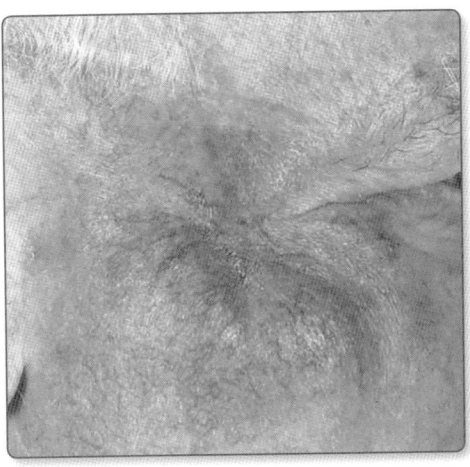

6.1 **Question**

What are the key features when examining a patient with the lesion shown in this figure?

Answer

- Size and site of lesion
- Clinical subtype
- Relationship to key anatomical structures, e.g. frontal branch of facial nerve
- Feasibility of design of local flap
- Dermatoscopy (Box A)

6.2 **Question**

What is the ideal margin?

Answer

- Refer to British Association of Dermatologists (BAD) guidelines
- Determined by subtype (Box B)
- A 4–5 mm margin will clear 95% of smaller BCCs (<20 mm)
- Larger BCCs (and morphoeic subtypes) require margins of 13–15 mm to achieve similar clearance rates

6.3 Question

How is a rhomboid flap designed?

Answer

- Also called Limberg flap, a rhomboid defect is created with internal angles of 60° and 120°
- Flap is designed as a limb off of one of the 120° angles
- Other line is drawn parallel to side of rhombus
- Combination of advancement and transposition moves the flap into the defect (Box C)
- This is a random pattern flap, with no named blood supply (as opposed to axial pattern flap, such as paramedian forehead flap)

6.4 Question

What is the role of Mohs micrographic surgery (MMS)?

Answer

- MMS may be used for higher risk lesions (Box D)
- Particularly useful for critical sites (e.g. periorbital) where considerable functional morbidity may be incurred

6.5 Question

What about the incompletely excised BCC?

Answer

- Recurrence rates for incompletely excised BCCs range from 30 to 41%
- Re-excision of incompletely excised tumours reveals residual tumour in only 55% of those examined using MMS
- Re-treatment should be re-excision, preferably using MMS, but radiotherapy may have a role in reducing recurrence rates
- High risk lesions and involved deep margins in particular should prompt consideration of re-excision

6.6 Question

What other treatment options are there besides surgical excision?

Answer

- Curettage and cautery
- Cryosurgery
- Photodynamic therapy (PDT)
- Carbon dioxide (CO_2) laser
- Topical immunotherapy with imiquimod
- Radiotherapy

Box A: The dermatoscope

- Dermatoscopy is a noninvasive diagnostic technique enabling magnification x 10–20
- It is used as an adjunct to clinical diagnosis to look for characteristics of BCC
- These include: ulceration; multiple gray-blue globules; maple leaf-like areas; spoke wheel areas; ulceration; and arborizing telangiectasia
- Sensitivity may be improved with the addition of reflectance confocal microscopy (RCM)

Box B: Basal cell carcinoma subtypes

- Low risk: nodular; superficial
- High risk: basosquamous; morphoeic; infiltrative; pigmented; micronodular
- Less commonly seen: metatypical; infundibulocystic; sclerosing; BCC with sebaceous differentiation

Box C: Local flap nomenclature

- Transposition: effectively where a portion of skin is moved around a pivot into an adjacent defect, e.g. rhomboid flap
- Rotation: commonly seen in scalp defect reconstruction, there is an semicircular arc of rotation to move adjacent skin based on a pedicle into the defect, e.g. O-to-S
- Interpolation: skin is raised on a pedicle and 'dropped' into a nearby (but not adjacent) defect with the pedicle bridging intact skin, e.g. paramedian forehead flap
- Advancement: skin is moved in laterally from an adjacent area, sometimes requiring the removal of Burrow's triangles, e.g. bilateral horizontal advancement flaps may be used at the temple

Box D: Indications for MMS

- Higher risk sites
- Larger tumours >20 mm in diameter
- Higher risk histological subtypes
- Poor clinical definition of tumour margins
- Recurrent lesions
- Perineural or perivascular involvement

Further reading

Longo C, Lallas A, Kyrgidis A, et al. Classifying distinct basal cell carcinoma subtype by means of dermatoscopy and reflectance confocal microscopy. J Am Acad Dermatol 2014; 71:716–724.

Telfer NR, Colver GB, Morton CA, et al. Guidelines for the management of basal cell carcinoma. Br J Dermatol 2008; 159:35–48.

Wozniak-Rito A, Zalaudek I, Rudnicka L. Dermoscopy of basal cell carcinoma. Clin Exp Dermatol 2018; 43:241–247.

Short case 7: Scalp reconstruction following squamous cell carcinoma

This patient has been brought in with a neglected nonhealing ulcer on the scalp.

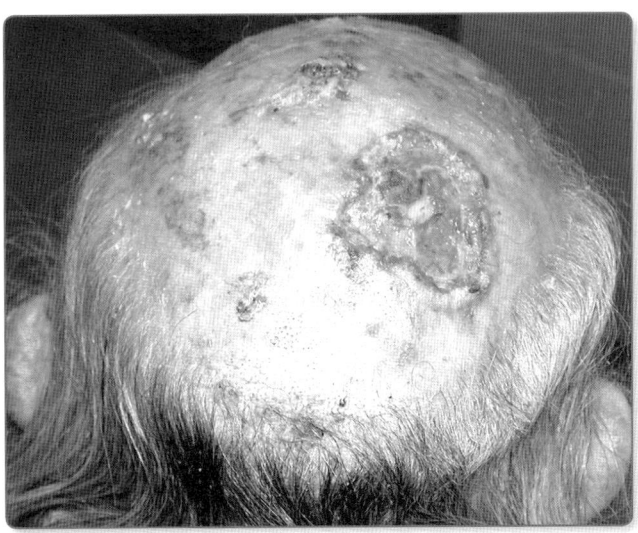

7.1 Question
What are the key features when examining a patient with the lesion shown in this figure?

Answer
- Assess dimensions of lesion
- Examine for regional lymphadenopathy: including level V and ipsilateral parotid

7.2 Question
What are the risk factors for cutaneous SCC?

Answer
- Exposure to UV light
- Ionising radiation exposure
- Chronic wounds, e.g. scars, burns
- Immunosuppression
- Precursor lesions, e.g. Bowen's disease (SCC in situ)
- Albinism, xeroderma pigmentosum
- Arsenic exposure

7.3 Question
What is the minimum histopathology dataset from an excision specimen?

Short case 7 Scalp reconstruction following squamous cell carcinoma

Answer

- Histological subtype (Box A)
- Degree of differentiation (grade)
- Tumour thickness
- Level of dermal invasion (Clark's level)
- Presence/absence perineural/lymphovascular invasion
- Margins

7.4 Question

How would you treat the lesion in the figure shown?

Answer

- Most commonly treated surgically
- Radiotherapy has comparable success rates for scalp lesions and may be indicated in some patients (Box B)

7.5 Question

What determines how you would reconstruct this relatively small scalp defect if treated surgically?

Answer

- Defect size
- Lesion risk: low or high (Box C)
- Presence of pericranium and whether it can be preserved
- In low risk smaller defects, local rotation/advancement flaps may be employed (e.g. pinwheel flap)
- Rotational flaps have the advantage of moving hair bearing skin

7.6 Question

What are the reconstructive options for a large defect?

Answer

- Skin graft (necessitates pericranium and recruits nonhair bearing skin)
- Dermal matrix substitutes (Box D)
- Tissue expanders
- Resurfacing with free flaps, e.g. latissimus dorsi and split thickness skin graft

7.7 Question

How should you treat the neck?

Answer

- No role for routine elective neck dissection in clinically N0 neck (approximately 5% of SCCs metastasise overall but proportion in higher risk tumours may be as high as 47%)

- Clinically palpable nodes should precipitate cross-sectional imaging and FNAC
- For N+ patients, dissection type guided by site of primary, e.g. II-V for P0/N+ posterior scalp lesion
- Parotidectomy required for P+ patients (parotid involved in 67-82%)

7.8 Question

What is the role of sentinel lymph node biopsy (SLNB) in cutaneous SCC?

Answer
- Increasing evidence that SLNB may have role in high risk SCC
- Evidence base lags behind that of melanoma
- Prospective sentinel node biopsy for high-risk SNIC trial is ongoing

---

Box A: Cutaneous SCC subtypes

- Subtypes have been classified by Cassarino et al.
- Low: HPV-associated SCC, tricholemmal carcinoma
- Intermediate: acantholytic, lymphoepithelioma-like
- High risk: adenosquamous carcinoma, malignant proliferating pilar tumours (strongly consider using Mohs)
- Undeterminate behavior

Box B: Indications for radiotherapy

- Radiotherapy may be used for primary treatment of cutaneous SCC
- Advantages include improved cosmetic outcome
- Comparable success rates to surgery in some regions, e.g. perioral
- Indications for adjuvant treatment in the scalp include nodal status >N1 and/or extracapsular spread

---

Box C: Higher risk lesions

- Tumours >2 cm diameter
- Tumours >4 mm depth or extending to Clark level V
- High-risk site involvement, e.g. ear, nonhair-bearing lip
- Poorly differentiated tumours (Broders grades 3 and 4)
- High-risk histological subtype
- Perineural and/or perivascular invasion
- Host immunosuppression
- Recurrent disease

> **Box D: Dermal matrix substitutes**
> - Dermal matrix substitutes support regeneration of host tissues (fibroblasts and capillary infiltrates)
> - They support skin grafting to full thickness scalp defects, potentially rivaling free flaps in terms of cost effectiveness and successful outcomes
> - Products available include porcine atelocollagen and silicone bilaminar sheet (Pelnac), and cross-linked bovine collagen and shark cartilage-derived chondroitin-6-sulfate (Integra)

Further reading

Cassarino DS, Derienzo DP, Barr RJ. Cutaneous squamous cell carcinoma: a comprehensive clinicopathologic classification – part two. J Cutan Pathol 2006; 33:261–279.

Gurney B, Newlands C. Management of regional metastatic disease in head and neck cutaneous malignancy. 1. Cutaneous squamous cell carcinoma. Br J Oral Maxillofac Surg 2014; 52: 294–300.

Motley RJ, Preston PW, Lawrence CM. Multi-professional guidelines for the management of the patient with primary cutaneous squamous cell carcinoma. Br J Dermatol 2002; 146:552–567.

Long case 8: Auricular reconstruction

The patient shown in the figure presents to the clinic.

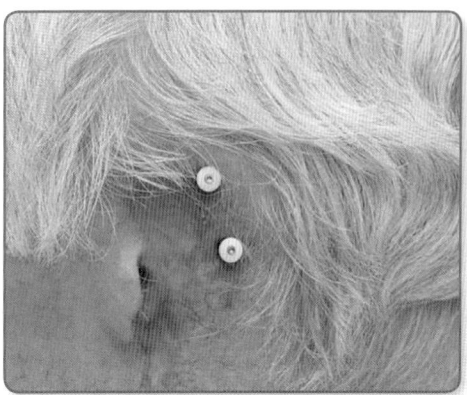

8.1 Question
What can you observe?

Answer
- Sub-total loss of left ear
- Two osseointegrated implants in situ
- Good skin quality around implants
- No evidence of infection

8.2 Question
What are the key points to ascertain in the history?

Answer
- Cause of loss: trauma, neoplasia, congenital
- Time since injury or resection
- Previous attempts at reconstruction
- Past medical history and drug history in relation to future surgery
- Social history: support, wearing of glasses

8.3 Question
What are the key points to ascertain in the examination?

Answer
- Defect size
- Remaining anatomical units (Box A)
- Remaining anatomical components: skin, cartilage
- Blood supply (Box B)
- Sensation (Box C)
- Skin: quality, signs of radiotherapy

- Implants: integration, position, evidence of infection
- Remaining face and scalp: other skin lesions
- Parotid
- Neck lumps

8.4 Question

Is there anything else you need to know before determining the management plan?

Answer

- Hearing
- Previous pathology report: diagnosis of lesion (Box D), resection margins, completeness of excision
- Patient preferences for reconstruction
- Previous radiotherapy (Box E)

8.5 Question

This patient originally presented with a 2 cm SCC. What would have been the treatment options?

Answer

- Smaller auricular defects are best approached by subunit
- Helical rim defects: Antia-Buch helical advancement flaps, tubed postauricular pedicle flaps (staged) or full thickness skin grafts (if perichondrium maintained)
- Conchal bowl defect: skin grafts, the 'revolving door' flap (pedicled skin from postauricular) or the postauricular island pedicled flap
- Helical rim, scapha and/or antihelix: wedge/star excisions, but larger defects may require more creative solutions such as staged postauricular flap with cartilage

8.6 Question

This patient clearly underwent pinnectomy. What are the reconstructive options?

Answer

- Broadly speaking, the options are autogenous or prosthetic

8.7 Question

How is autogenous reconstruction undertaken?

Answer

- Uses 6–9th costochondral cartilage
- Staged reconstructive approach
- The soft tissue covering comes from either tissue expansion or a TPFF with overlying skin graft

- Porous polyethylene frameworks have been used for total ear reconstruction, but have been associated with high extrusion rates

8.8 Question

Why might this patient have had prosthetic rehabilitation instead?

Answer

- The success rates of implant retained prostheses are high
- This is especially in irradiated bone (Box C)

8.9 Question

What design would you choose?

Answer

- Plan in conjunction with prosthetist
- Commonly place three implants linked by a bar
- Magnet-retained prostheses tend to have lower patient satisfaction

---

Box A: Anatomy of the pinna

- Helical rim
- Superior crus
- Scapha
- Antihelix
- Concha
- Triangular fossa
- Cymbum concha
- Root of helix
- External auditory meatus
- Tragus
- Cavum concha
- Intertragal notch
- Antitragus
- Lobule

Box B: Blood supply of the pinna

- Posterior auricular artery
- Occipital artery
- Superficial temporal artery

Box C: Sensory supply to the ear

- Greater auricular nerve (C2–C3) to the lower half of the pinna
- Lesser occipital nerve (C2) to the medial aspect of the superior half
- Auriculotemporal nerve (CN Vc) to the lateral aspect of the superior half
- Auricular branch of the vagus nerve, also known as Arnold's nerve (CN X) to the auditory canal and concha

Box D: Commonest skin cancers to affect the auricle

- Squamous cell carcinoma (50–60%)
- Basal cell carcinoma (30–40%)
- Melanoma

Box E: Implants and radiation

- Placement of implants in irradiated bone is detrimental to the chances of a successful outcome (94–99% versus 58–91% reported)
- The question remains of placement in relation to timing of radiotherapy
- A large single centre study demonstrated no impact of the timing of radiotherapy on implant success in a cohort including auricular, orbital and nasal implants (both 6% failure rate)
- Cortical bone is at a premium in this region and 3–4 mm Cochlear Vistafix implants are often used
- Implants are placed at 1:30, 3 o'clock and 4:30 in the left ear
- In the right ear they were placed at 10:30, 9 o'clock and 7:30
- A CT scan was used for reference in conjunction with a maxillofacial prosthetist

Further reading

Elledge R, Chaggar J, Knapp N, et al. Craniofacial implants at a single centre 2005-2015. Br J Oral Maxillofac Surg 2017; 55:242–245.

Menick FJ. Reconstruction of the ear after tumour excision. Clin Plast Surg 1990; 17:405–415.

Sherris DA, Larrabee WF Jr. Principles of Facial Reconstruction: A Subunit Approach to Cutaneous Repair, 2nd Edition. Thieme, New York 2009.

Chapter 5

Facial trauma

SHORT CASES

1. Isolated nasal fracture
2. Anterior table frontal sinus fracture
3. Penetrating neck injury
4. NOE complex fracture
5. Infected mandible fracture
6. Ballistic mandible fracture
7. Edentulous mandible fracture
8. Orbital floor fracture repair
9. Mandibular condyle fracture
10. Zygomaticomaxillary complex fracture

LONG CASE

11. Panfacial fractures

Short case 1: Isolated nasal fracture

This 15-year-old woman shown in the figure has been allegedly assaulted.

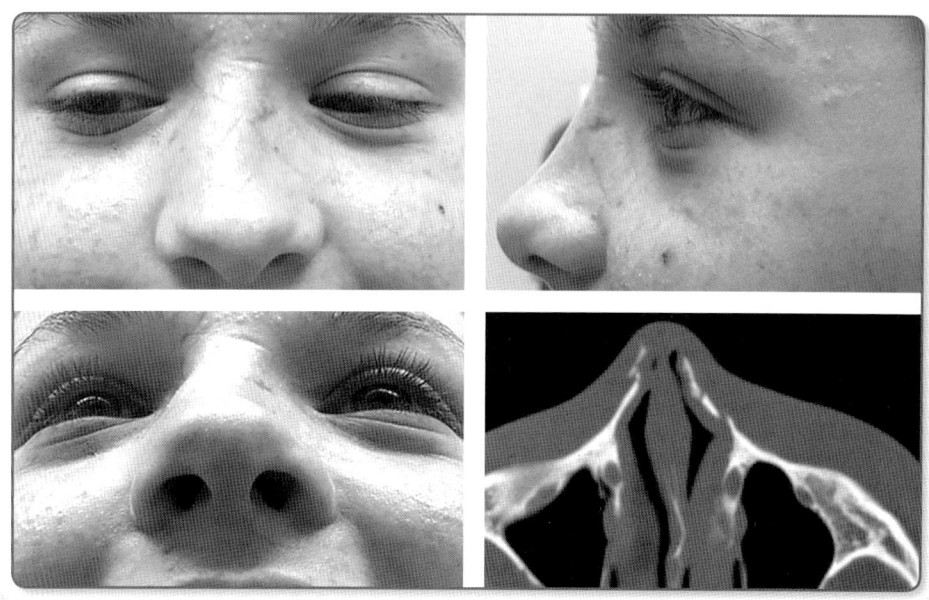

1.1 **Question**

How would you assess this patient?

Answer

- Requires tailored history and examination

1.2 **Question**

What are the key points in the history?

Answer

- Time post injury
- Altered appearance: deviation, flattening
- Epistaxis
- Previous facial trauma or surgery
- Numbness of cheek: may indicate a naso-orbital-ethmoidal (NOE) fracture
- Other injuries: head injury, midface fracture.

1.3 **Question**

What are the key points in the examination?

Answer

Inspection:
- End of bed: asymmetry, lacerations, other injuries

- Front: deviation at upper third (nasal bones), rhinion (junction), lower two-thirds (lateral cartilages), increased nostril show
- Side: dorsal collapse, loss of tip projection
- Worms eye: septal deviation (cartilaginous and/or bony)
- Speculum: septal haematoma, airway patency

Palpation:
- Pain over nasal dorsum, infraorbital rim
- Occlude each nostril in turn getting patient to breath in and out

1.4 Question
Would you request any imaging?

Answer
- Neither plain films or CT imaging are required for isolated nasal fractures
- CT may be required should other injuries such as a NOE be suspected (Box A)

1.5 Question
How would you tread this nasal fracture?

Answer
- Closed (LA with sedation or GA) (Box B)
- Early open
- Delayed open: waiting for 3–4 months to operate electively only appropriate if other reasons such as patient's medical condition preclude an operation

1.6 Question
You agree to perform closed surgery. What are the potential risks for the patient?

Answer
- Septal deviation: as scar matures resulting in poor nasal flow
- Dorsal collapse recurs: saddle nose deformity
- Need for repeat surgery
- Restricted growth: in female patients <16 years old the nasal septum still a growth centre for anterior maxillary growth

1.7 Question
After 3 months she still has asymmetry. What do you suggest?

Answer
- An open septorhinoplasty
- Septoplasty often requires removal of deviated part of quadrangular cartilage and perpendicular plate of ethmoid bone or vomer
- Osteotomies of nasal bones may be followed up by dorsal grafting with septal, conchal or rib cartilage
- A spreader graft may be required to improve any internal nasal valve obstruction

Box A: The use of CT for nasal bone fractures
- The gold standard for determining the degree of comminution of nasal bones
- Demonstrates deviation of nasal bones and cartilaginous septum
- May show propagation towards the orbit (i.e. NOE fracture)

Box B: One method for closed reduction of an isolated nasal fracture
- Haemostatic pledgets inserted into the nostrils for 10 minutes
- Local anaesthetic blocks
- Walsham forceps to straighten the septum
- Howarths to elevate nasal bones
- Each nostril is packed for a week and the patient given oral antibiotics
- A splint is sometimes placed on the nasal dorsum

Further reading

Mondin V, Rinaldo A, Ferlito A. Management of nasal bone fractures. Am J Otolaryngol 2005; 26:181–185.

Short case 2: Anterior table frontal sinus fracture

This patient has returned to clinic 3 months following a road traffic collision.

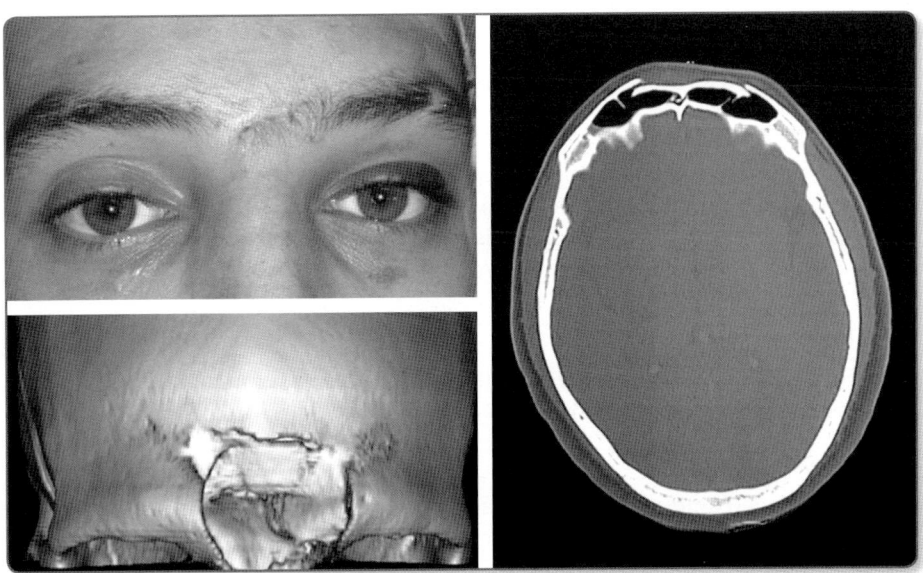

2.1 Question

What are the key points in the examination when the patient first presented in the emergency department?

Answer
- Overlying laceration: potential communication with underlying fracture
- Deformity: difficult to assess when swollen
- Neurological: Glasgow Coma Score must be recorded, assess for cerebrospinal fluid (CSF) leak (Box A), forehead sensation
- Eyes: telecanthus, visual acuity, range of movements, globe position
- Other injuries

2.2 Question

What can you see on these images?

Answer

3D reformatted image:
- Supraorbital and NOE fractures, probably involving the frontal sinus

Axial CT slice at level of frontal sinus:
- Anterior table: comminuted and displaced
- Posterior table: intact, no intracranial air or blood
- Floor: cannot assess frontonasal ducts, pneumatised with no fluid level

- Need to review all slices in all planes
- Liaise with neurosurgery department regarding posterior wall damage and intracranial injury

2.3 Question

How can you tell if the frontonasal duct is patent?

Answer

- Preoperative: CT showing fracture passing through it (although may still be patent), or fluid level (blockage)
- Intraoperative: direct visualisation, blue dye
- Postoperative: mucocele, recurrent sinusitis

2.4 Question

How would you manage the frontal sinus injuries, assuming there was no posterior wall involvement on CT?

Answer

- Displaced anterior sinus wall fracture evident that optimally requires treatment for cosmetic reasons (Box B)
- Sinus may potentially communicate with skin via overlying laceration producing an open fracture
- Explore laceration and clean under local anaesthetic
- If it does not communicate with fracture, laceration can be closed and further treatment deferred
- If laceration communicates with underlying fracture arguments exist for both early and delayed repair (Box C)

2.5 Question

What further treatment would you perform?

Answer

- Most anterior wall fractures treated surgically although transnasal endoscopic fixation is used
- Coronal flap (laceration extension unlikely to provide suitable access)
- Assess frontonasal duct and posterior wall for damage
- Fracture fixation with low profile miniplates
- Debride and suture laceration if not done already

2.6 Question

What would you do if you felt the frontonasal duct was obstructed?

Answer

- If posterior wall not affected re-establish patency via endoscopic-guided drainage tube

- If this is not possible, or there is posterior wall involvement then manage by obliteration or cranialisation
- 3% of cases with obstructed frontonasal ducts treated conservatively resulted in complications

2.7 Question

When you see the patient in clinic today there is still a noticeable dent. How would you manage this?

Answer

- Wait 6 weeks for swelling to fully subside
- Request CT scan to assess defect size
- Reaccess coronal flap: titanium plate, Medpor or PEEK implant
- Endoscopic access through hairline: same as above
- Injectable filler: autologous fat, calcium hydroxyapatite or poly-L-lactic acid

2.8 Question

At the time of initial surgery, the neurosurgeon felt the patient was unlikely to achieve a good outcome. Would you still proceed with the operation?

Answer

- Strong body of evidence to support conservative management of even displaced posterior wall fractures
- Majority of displaced frontal sinus fractures are treated due to risk of long-term complications (Box D)
- Some patients with very poor initial neurological prognosis do improve and performing surgery at later date has greater risk than early surgery

---

Box A: Testing for CSF leaks

Clinical signs:
- Persistent rhinorrhoea
- Halo sign

Tests:
- Beta-2 transferrin (Tau protein)
- CT or MR cisternography: determines exact location

Box B: Indications for surgery in frontal sinus fractures

- Anterior table: cosmetic defect, open to skin
- Posterior table: displacement >table width/5 mm (likely CSF leak), proven CSF leak, meningitis, pneumocephalus
- Floor: obstruction of either frontonasal duct

> **Box C: Early versus delayed repair of open frontal sinus fractures**
>
> Argument for early:
> - This constitutes an 'open fracture'
> - Such fractures are at a higher risk of infection unless cleaned and fixed
>
> Argument for delayed repair:
> - If the wound breaks down it could result in a fistula
> - By closing the laceration and waiting for a week before surgery it gives the skin time to heal before undertaking a coronal flap

> **Box D: Potential complications of frontal sinus fractures**
>
> - Anterior: cosmetic defect, overlying skin fistulation
> - Floor: mucocele
> - Posterior: persistent CSF leak leading to meningitis or brain abscess

Further reading

Choi M, Li Y, Shapiro SA, et al. A 10-year review of frontal sinus fractures: clinical outcomes of conservative management of posterior table fractures. Plast Reconstr Surg 2012; 130:399–406.

Gerbino G, Roccia F, Benech A, et al. Analysis of 158 frontal sinus fractures: current surgical management and complications. J Craniomaxillofac Surg 2000; 28:133–139.

Rodriguez ED, Stanwix MG, Nam AJ, et al. Twenty-six-year experience treating frontal sinus fractures: a novel algorithm based on anatomical fracture pattern and failure of conventional techniques. Plast Reconstr Surg 2008; 122:1850–1866.

Sakas DE, Beale DJ, Ameen AA, et al. Compound anterior cranial base fractures: classification using computerized tomography scanning as a basis for selection of patients for dural repair. J Neurosurg 1998; 88:471–477.

Short case 3: Penetrating neck injury

This patient shown in the figure returns to clinic having previously suffered a penetrating neck injury.

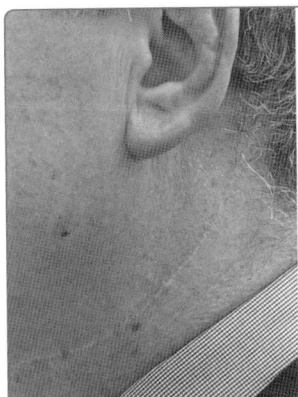
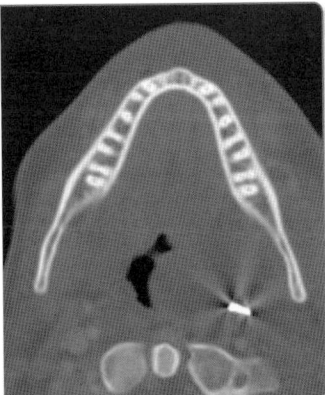

3.1 Question

What are the key points in the history?

Answer

- Mechanism of injury: projectile, blade, blunt
- Investigations and surgery performed
- Medical and drug history
- Complications of trauma or surgery (Box A)

3.2 Question

How would you examine the patient in clinic?

Answer

- Entry and/or exit wound location(s)
- Incision: location, neck zone (Box B)
- Nerves: marginal mandibular, hypoglossal, lingual, accessory
- Swallowing
- Talking

3.3 Question

This patient originally presented to the emergency department with a large gaping zone 2 entry wound that was packed with a dressing. How would you have managed them?

Answer

- ATLS principles
- Anaesthetic input and inform theatre coordinator
- If likely to have breached platysma do not remove dressing to inspect further

3.4 Question

This is the scan the patient had taken in the emergency department on their first visit. What can you ascertain from the scan?

Answer

- CT angiogram in axial section: above lower border of mandible (Zone 3)
- Foreign object with high signal intensity: probably metallic
- Swelling of soft tissue causing reduction of airway diameter
- Object in close proximity to carotid arteries and jugular veins, but no obvious damage or blood
- Need to review other slices

3.5 Question

How would you have ascertained signs of damage to nonvascular structures, such as the aerodigestive tract, from this CT?

Answer

- Aerodigestive injury can be difficult to diagnose on CT alone
- If symptoms of aerodigestive injury present then flexible nasendoscopy required
- Nasendoscopy should be performed immediately prior to theatre as it may induce coughing and further bleeding

3.6 Question

The patient was haemodynamically stable with no hard signs. Would you have explored surgically?

Answer

- Surgery should be performed on unstable patients or those in which hard signs are present (Box D)
- Access to injuries in zones 1 and 3 can be challenging
- Stable patients with isolated active haemorrhage should be discussed with interventional radiology if facilities exist (Box D)

3.7 Question

This patient was injured in an explosion and taken straight to theatre. Why was the incision shown in the figure used?

Answer

- Access to concurrent mandibular fracture
- Extension of cut made by foreign object originally
- Access to trachea or oesophagus to repair injury

- If haemodynamically stable then CT angiogram (Box C)
- If unstable from neck wound then straight to theatre for exploration

3.8 Question

In theatre the wound may have damaged the trachea and oesophagus. What would you do?

Answer

- In absence of evidence of damage on CT and lack of symptoms then do not formally explore
- Endoscope trachea and oesophagus
- If no damage seen, perform water-soluble contrast swallow postoperatively

---

Box A: Consequences of damage to cervical structures

- Vascular: exsanguination
- Neurological: brachial plexus, ischaemic stroke
- Airway: hypoxia, respiratory arrest
- Oesophagus: dysphagia, tracheo-oesophageal fistula

Box B: Neck zones in penetrating trauma

- Zone I: suprasternal notch to cricoid cartilage
- Zone II: cricoid cartilage to angle of mandible
- Zone III: angle of mandible to base of skull

Box C: Clinical 'hard signs' of penetrating neck injury warranting immediate surgical exploration

- Vascular: bleeding not amenable to pressure, expanding haematoma, bruit or thrill
- Aerodigestive injury: subcutaneous emphysema, dyspnoea, air bubbling, pain over trachea, altered voice, hematemesis, haemoptysis

---

Box D: Interventional radiology options

- Transarterial embolisation: effective in treating active haemorrhage to smaller vessels, especially if the collateral circulation allows for vessel's sacrifice
- Endovascular stent placement: more appropriate for injuries involving large and medium sized vessels that must remain patent

---

Box E: Access incision choices approaches to the neck

- Anterior sternocleidomastoid incision
- Anterior sternocleidomastoid incision with sternotomy extension
- Collar incision
- Visor incision

Further reading

Breeze J, Powers D. Penetrating neck injury. In: Ballistic Trauma, 4th Edition. Springer 2017.

Nowicki J, Stew B, Ooi E. Penetrating neck injuries: a guide to evaluation and management. Ann R Coll Surg Engl 2018; 100:6–11.

Short case 4: NOE complex fracture

This patient shown in the figure has been transferred from another hospital with untreated midfacial fractures.

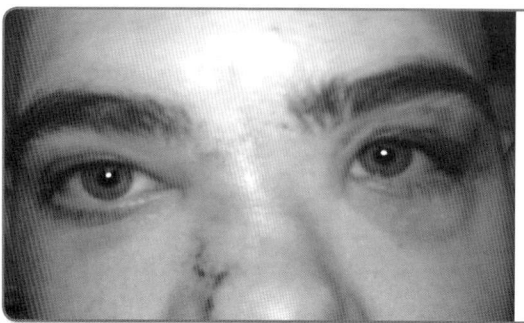
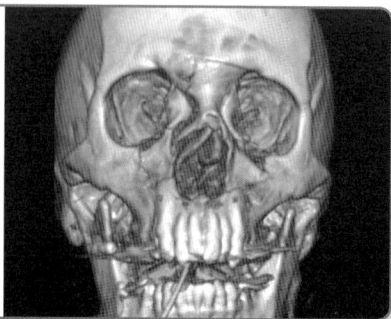

4.1 Question

What are the key points in the history?

Answer

- Time since injury
- Altered appearance
- Previous facial injuries and surgery
- Other injuries to face or remaining body, e.g. traumatic brain injury
- Eyes: altered vision
- Cheek sensation: cheek, teeth
- Nose: epistaxis and nasal drip (CSF)
- Occlusion
- Past medical and drug history
- Social history, including smoking

4.2 Question

What are the key points in the examination?

Answer

- Inspection: front, sides, above
- Palpate bones
- Sensation: cheek, nose, teeth
- Transverse width: facial fifths, intercanthal distance (30–35 mm, mean 33 mm)
- Nose: flattened bridge (saddle), nasal drip (CSF)
- Eyes: range of movements, enophthalmos, epiphora (nasolacrimal duct damage)
- Intraoral: occlusion, teeth damage

4.3 Question

Examination demonstrates telecanthus. Can you comment on the patient's images?

Answer

- 3D reformatted CT scan showing complex comminuted midfacial fractures
- NOE complex: crumpled with reduced AP projection and increased transverse dimension
- Frontal sinus: two large minimally-displaced fragments affecting supra orbital areas bilaterally
- Infraorbital rims: bilateral and very displaced on left side

4.4 Question

How would you manage the patient further?

Answer

- Liaise with neurosurgery and ophthalmology but try to treat patient within 10 days
- Frontal sinus: rule out posterior wall fracture and damage to frontal nasal duct
- Eye: range of movements, acuity, visual fields, nasolacrimal duct for damage

4.5 Question

Would any classifications help guide your treatment?

Answer

- Markowitz's classification reflects the importance of medial canthal tendon in guiding treatment (Box A)
- In the CT scan shown in the figure, the tendon is attached to a displaced large fragment, making it a Markowitz and Manson 1 (Box A)
- The fragment could be plated to the adjacent frontal bone (Box B)

4.6 Question

How would you access the fractures assuming the frontal sinus was only fractured anteriorly?

Answer

- Coronal flap: frontal sinus, nasal bridge
- Transconjunctival post-septal incision: orbital rim and floor
- Transcaruncular extension: medial orbital wall and canthal tendon
- Intraoral vestibular incisions: if required to access nasomaxillary buttress and piriform ring

4.7 Question

How would you reduce and fix the fractures?

Answer

- No generally accepted sequence but many use the 8 steps suggested by Ellis (Box C)
- Frontal sinus: reduce and fix individual fragments with miniplates
- Bone attached to left medial canthal tendon: plate to frontal bone (coronal flap), maxilla (intraoral) and infraorbital rim (transconjunctival) (Box D)
- Nasal bones: elevate nasal bones and plate to adjacent bones, straighten septum, augment dorsum if required with outer cortex calvarial bone graft
- Medial and floor of orbit: preformed plate or patient-specific implant

4.8 Question

How do you manage potential damage to the nasolacrimal duct?

Answer

- Preoperatively: examine individual CT slices
- Intraoperatively: examine duct orifice for injury. Only if grossly damaged, should cannulation and stenting be considered (Box E)
- Postoperatively: if epiphora occurs, perform CT dacrocystogram and if necessary dacryocystorhinostomy

---

Box A: Markowitz and Manson classification of nasoethmoidal orbital fractures

Based upon the insertion of the medial canthal tendon into the frontal process of the maxilla:
- 1: large fragment, tendon attached
- 2: comminuted fragments, tendon attached
- 3: comminuted fragments, tendon not attached

Box B: Suggested treatment

- Undisplaced: no treatment required
- Markowitz 1: three-point fixation at nasofrontal junction, infraorbital rim, and piriform rim
- Markowitz 2: wire the fragment containing the MCT to the contralateral side of the nose
- Markowitz 3: reattach MCL with nonabsorbable suture

Box C: Sequencing of treatment

- Exposure: usually coronal flap
- Identification of the tendon bearing fragment
- Reduce/reconstruct medial aspect of lower orbital rim
- Reconstruct medial orbital wall
- Reduce septal fractures or displacement
- Transnasal canthopexy if required
- Doral nasal reconstruction
- Soft tissue readaptation

Box D: Transnasal canthopexy

- Two parallel holes are placed in the bone attached to the medial canthus
- Holes are made superior and posterior to the original position
- Drill from contralateral nasofrontal region and pass the wire from there and back
- Risk of breaking bone when wire tightened

Box E: Management of nasolacrimal duct injury

- Medial canthal tendon overlies the lacrimal fossa
- Even in severe NOE fractures the nasolacrimal duct system is rarely damaged
- Damage can be difficult to identify preoperatively
- CT dacrocystogram uses conjunctival application of contrast medium
- Epiphora may reflect temporary blockage due to inflammation
- Damaged ducts are generally managed conservatively
- Only if grossly damaged should it be cannulated and stented
- Only 5–10% of patients with severe NOE fractures eventually require dacryocystorhinostomy

Further reading

Ellis E. Sequencing treatment for naso-orbito-ethmoid fractures. J Oral Maxillofac Surg 1993; 51:543–558.

Gruss JS, Hurwitz JJ, Nik NA, et al. The pattern and incidence of nasolacrimal injury in naso-orbital-ethmoid fractures: the role of delayed assessment and dacryocystorhinostomy. Br J Plast Surg 1985; 38:116–121.

Markowitz BL, Manson PN, Sargent L, et al. Management of the medial canthal tendon in nasoethmoid orbital fractures: the importance of the central fragment in classification and treatment. Plast Reconstr Surg 1991; 87:843–853.

Short case 5: Infected mandible fracture

The patient shown in the figure returns to trauma clinic with problems after having their mandible fixed 3 months ago.

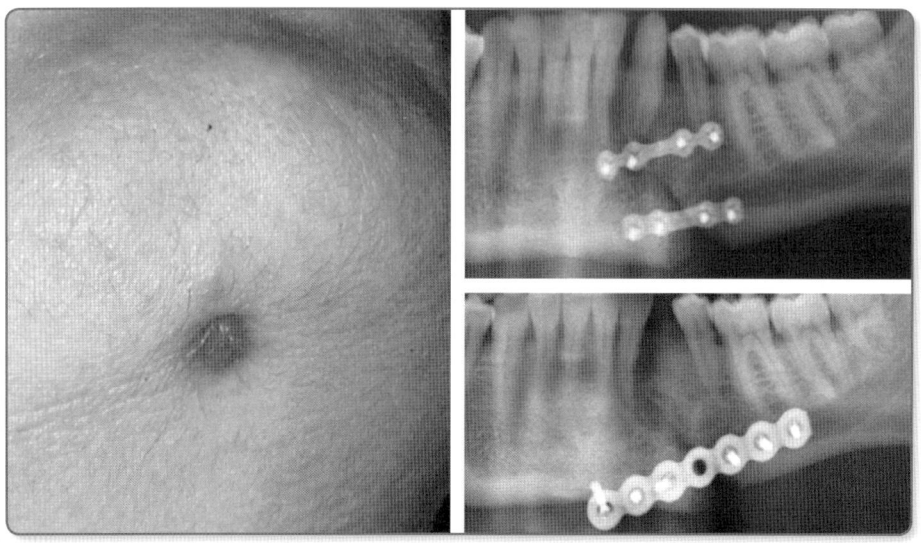

5.1 Question
What are the key points in the history?

Answer
- Current symptoms: pain, occlusion, numbness, mobility, infection
- Previous treatment: fixation type, surgical approach, complications
- Medical health and drug history (Box A)
- Social history: smoking, compliance with soft diet

5.2 Question
What are the key points in the examination?

Answer

Extraoral:
- Swelling
- Cutaneous sinus
- Mouth opening
- Lip numbness

Intraoral:
- Fracture site and teeth mobility
- Wound dehiscence and plate exposure
- Occlusion
- Oral hygiene

5.3 **Question**

There is a cutaneous sinus under the chin. How would you manage the patient from here?

Answer
- Diagnosis: probable infection and nonunion at fracture site
- OPG: plate position, prognosis of teeth
- CT: extent of necrosis, evidence of osteomyelitis, sinus path

5.4 **Question**

What can you ascertain from this upper radiographic image of the patient taken in clinic?

Answer
- OPG demonstrating left parasymphysis fracture involving canine
- Repaired with two straight plates that appear mono cortical
- Eburnated bone ends with gap between them
- Signs are suggestive of inadequate fracture reduction

5.5 **Question**

How would you manage the patient further?

Answer
- Patient requires revision surgery
- Re-access fracture site through transcutaneous approach
- Removal of existing plates and screws
- Debridement necrotic bone or interposing soft tissue
- Remove teeth of poor prognosis
- Rigid immobilisation with load bearing osteosynthesis (Box B)
- Heavy profile noncompression locking plate
- Three locking screws at least 1 cm either side of fracture site
- Fistulectomy
- Adjuncts (Box C)

5.6 **Question**

Would you bone graft at the same time?

Answer
- Yes, a nonvascularised autologous bone graft can be placed in active infection
- Evidence for bone substitutes unclear and probably best to wait 3 months

5.7 **Question**

Can you comment on this postoperative image?

Answer
- OPG of the same patient showing a 7-hole plate with 3 screws either side of fracture site
- Plate not at lower border
- Most proximal screw potentially in the IA canal
- Poor plate position may be due to procedure having been performed via intraoral approach

5.8 Question
How would you follow up this patient?

Answer
- Every 2 weeks to ensure intraoral and skin fistula healing
- OPG radiograph in 4 weeks should show new bone formation
- Healing may take several weeks

Box A: Risk factors for nonunion in mandible fractures

Fracture factors:
- Atrophic mandible height
- Infection
- Devitalised teeth
- Inadequate or poorly placed fixation

Patient factors:
- Immunosuppression: systemic (e.g. diabetes), and iatrogenic (e.g. steroids)
- Poor oral hygiene
- Smoking
- Noncompliance with soft diet
- Further trauma

Box B: Broad treatment options for mandibular nonunion

- Rigid fixation
- External fixation
- Maxillary mandibular fixation (MMF): success rates tend to be poor due to patient compliance

---

Box C: Adjuncts to healing in mandibular nonunion

Systemic:
- Antibiotics

Fracture site:
- Bone graft
- Gentamicin powder/beads

Disputed benefit:
- Hyperbaric oxygen
- Bone morphogenic protein

Further reading

Alpert B, Kushner GM, Tiwana PS. Contemporary management of infected mandibular fractures. Craniomaxillofac Trauma Reconstr 2008; 1:25–29.

Benson PD, Marshall MK, Engelstad ME, et al. The use of immediate bone grafting in the reconstruction of clinically infected mandibular fractures: bone grafts in the presence of pus. J Oral Maxillofac Surg 2006; 64:122–126.

Mehra P, Van Heukelom E, Cottrell DA. Rigid internal fixation of infected mandibular fractures. J Oral Maxillofac Surg 2009; 67:1046–1051.

Short case 6: Ballistic mandible fracture

The patient shown in this figure has returned to trauma clinic today.

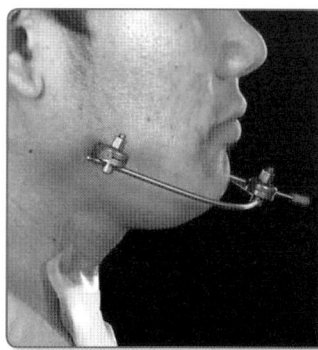
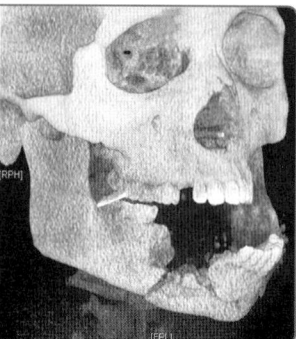

6.1 Question

What can you can see from the left image and what is it used for?

Answer

- Postoperative patient with a mandibular external fixator in situ
- Dressing over a tracheostomy site
- Potential indications in trauma described in Box A

6.2 Question

This patient sustained a facial gunshot wound (GSW). How would you examine him?

Answer

- End of bed: general health, other injuries, gastric feeding tube
- Extraoral: pin stability and erythema, scars indicative of entry or exit sites
- Intraoral: occlusion, missing teeth, ridge shape and height
- Signs of high energy transfer: avulsive tissue loss

6.3 Question

You are shown the image on the right. What can you see?

Answer

- Three-dimensional reformat of a CT scan
- Probably taken shortly after injury
- Grossly comminuted mandible
- Avulsive bone defect and lack of bony continuity on right side
- No obvious retained bullet

6.4 Question
How would you manage this patient in the emergency department?

Answer
- ABCDE approach (Box B)
- Orally intubate
- Straight to theatre if uncontrolled bleeding or unable to secure airway
- CT scan if stable

6.5 Question
This is the patient's only injury and there was no acute airway or bleeding. What would you do in theatre?

Answer
- Surgical tracheostomy
- Debride soft tissue injury
- Stabilise but consider not internally fixing the mandible fracture acutely if signs of high energy transfer (Box C)

6.6 Question
The bullet fragmented prior to exit and a 5-mm piece is retained. Would you remove it?

Answer
- In acute setting remove foreign bodies if you can find them without causing damage
- In longer term remove if they are causing problems

6.7 Question
The fragment is located in the parotid gland. How could you remove it?

Answer
- Dissection through overlying scar if present
- Assistance with intraoperative CT or navigation
- Formal parotidectomy

6.8 Question
What are your longer-term options?

Answer
- Leave external fixator or IMF for 6 weeks then assess fragment union
- Some clinicians perform ORIF after a week or so once vascularity likely to have improved
- Soft tissue surgery: serial debridement, scar release, vestibuloplasty
- Bone augmentation (Box D)

> **Box A: Potential indications for an external fixator in the trauma setting**
> - Severe comminution
> - Wound contamination
> - Avulsion and loss of hard tissue at the time of injury
> - Contraindications to ORIF

> **Box B: Broad management options for a facial GSW in the ED setting**
> - Airway: anaesthetic support for early intubation – +/- surgical airway
> - Cervical spine immobilisation: 10% of facial GSWs have an associated cervical spinal fracture
> - Breathing: bullets may ricochet and the wound tract is unpredictable
> - Circulation: fluid resuscitation with blood products if necessary
> - Disability: GCS should be assessed prior to intubation if possible
> - Exposure: other injuries

> **Box C: Options for stabilisation of mandible fractures due to gunshot wounds**
> - Intermaxillary fixation: likely to necessitate tracheostomy
> - Internal fixation through intraoral approach: not for high energy transfer wounds
> - Internal fixation through extraoral approach: not if risk of further devitalisation
> - External fixation

> **Box D: Options for augmenting an avulsive mandibular segment**
> - Vascularised graft
> - Nonvascularised graft
> - Titanium mesh with bone substitute
> - Distraction: intra or extraoral

Further reading

Breeze J, Parmar S. High-energy ballistic injuries to the face. In: Challenging Concepts in Oral and Maxillofacial Surgery, Oxford University Press 2016.

Short case 7: Edentulous mandible fracture

The patient in the figure is awaiting treatment of their mandible fracture.

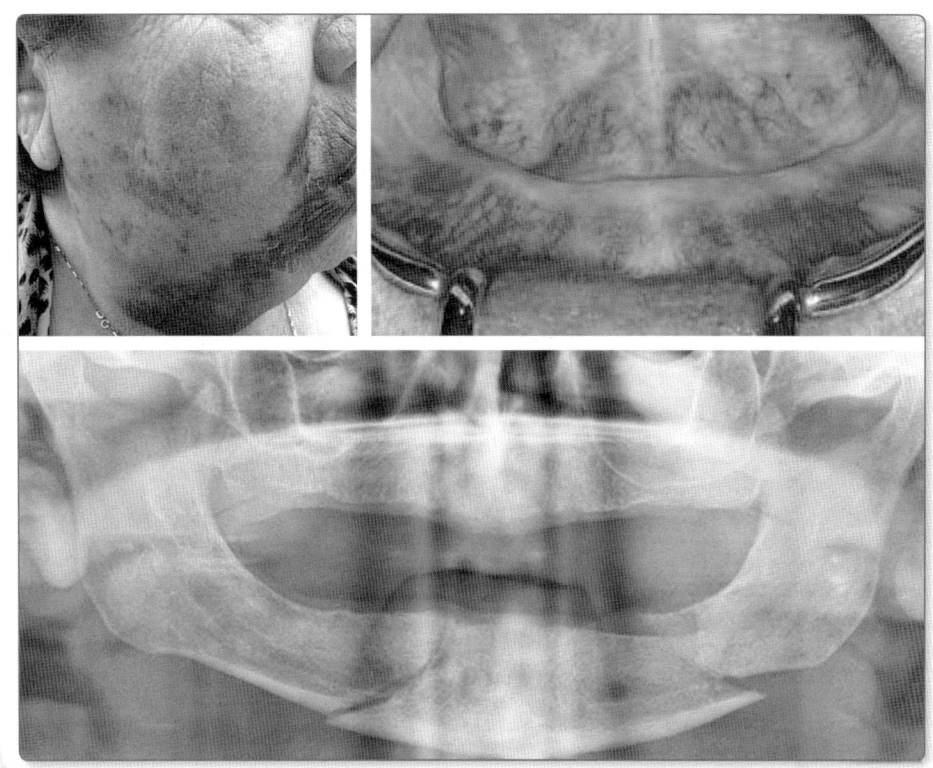

7.1 Question

How would you assess the patient?

Answer

- Patient has cutaneous and mucosal bruising consistent with bilateral edentulous mandible fracture as demonstrated in OPG radiograph
- Assessment in nonacute setting would comprise tailored history, examination and review of pertinent imaging

7.2 Question

What are the key points in the history?

Answer

- Age of injury
- Wearing dentures
- Medical comorbidities: particular those predisposing to pathological fracture
- Medications: particularly those pertinent to surgery
- Social support postdischarge

7.3 Question
What are the key points in the examination?

Answer
- Lip sensation
- Fracture mobility
- Mucosal tears overlying fracture

7.4 Question
What imaging would you request and how would it guide your management?

Answer
- Plain radiographs: most clinicians supplement OPG radiographs with PA mandible to enable identification of fracture displacement, bone height (Box A), and bone pathology (cyst, metastasis, etc.)
- CT: usually only required for suspected premorbid bone pathology, or construction of splints

7.5 Question
There is no intraoral injury but the fracture is grossly unstable and painful. How would you treat this patient?

Answer
As the image demonstrates a good height of bone with no significant trauma to the mucosa, many surgeons would attempt intraoral approach with load-sharing ostesynthesis

7.6 Question
What other options are available?

Answer
- Instability of fracture necessitates intervention (Box B)
- Conservative management not appropriate in this case

7.7 Question
How would you treat a displaced unstable fracture of a mandible of only 10 mm height?

Answer
- Luhr type 2 and 3 fractures should be treated by load-bearing osteosynthesis
- Intraoral approach risks devitalising bone, therefore transcutaneous approach recommended
- Displaced fracture may be challenging to reduce through transmucosal approach alone, so transcutaneous approach would be indicated

7.8 Question
How would you access the mandible through a transcutaneous approach?

Answer

- Local anaesthetic infiltration
- Marking of submandibular cutaneous incision two finger widths below mandible
- Incise through skin, platysma and deep cervical fascia
- Dissect under deep cervical fascia superiority onto mandible
- Incise through periosteum directly into fracture

7.9 Question

Where would you expect the mandibular branch of the facial nerve to be?

Answer

- Anterior to the facial vessels (around antegonial notch) the nerve is below the mandible in 20% of patients
- Located on undersurface of platysma

Box A: Luhr classification of edentulous mandible fractures

Utilises the vertical height of the mandible at its narrowest point.
- Type 1: 16–20 mm
- Type 2: 11–15 mm
- Type 3: 10 mm or less

Box B: Treatment options for an edentulous mandible fracture

- Nonsurgical: soft diet
- Circummandibular wiring or screw fixation of existing denture
- Circummandibular wiring or screw fixation of a fabricated Gunning splint (of little clinical use in modern practice)
- Closed reduction with transmucosal plating (very specific clinical criteria required and ensuring plate is not directly abutting mucosa is essential)
- Open reduction with submucosal plating
- Open reduction through transcutaneous approach

Box C: Matching the Luhr classification to methods of open reduction

- Luhr 1: load sharing osteosynthesis, usually intraoral
- Luhr 2 or 3: load bearing osteosynthesis, by either transmucosal plating or transcutaneous approach
- Bone grafting as described by Luhr for grade 3 bone heights are in practice rarely used

---

Further reading

Luhr HG, Reidick T, Merten HA. Results of treatment of fractures of the atrophic edentulous mandible by compression plating: a retrospective evaluation of 84 consecutive cases. J Oral Maxillofac Surg 1996; 54:250–254.

Nasser M, Fedorowicz Z, Ebadifar A. Management of the fractured edentulous atrophic mandible. Cochrane Database Syst Rev 2007; 24:CD006087.

Short case 8: Orbital floor fracture repair

This patient attends trauma clinic following orbital surgery.

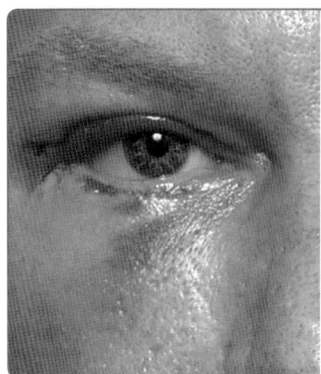
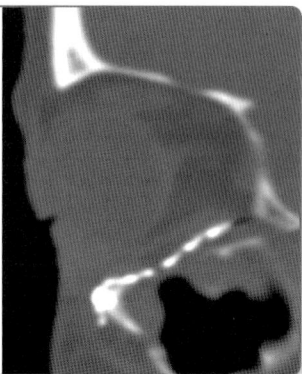

8.1 Question
What are the key points in the history?

Answer
- Time from initial injury to surgery
- Time postsurgery to current follow-up
- Type of surgery performed
- Symptoms: altered/double vision, numbness
- Symptoms present before surgery
- Other injuries
- General medical health and drug history
- Social history: smoking, occupation (e.g. lorry driver)

8.2 Question
The patient complains of diplopia. What are the key points in the examination?

Answer
- Surgical incision sites
- Globe position
- Pupil reactivity
- Cover test: monocular or binocular diplopia
- Range of movements
- Exophthalmometer

8.3 Question
How soon would you repair an isolated orbital floor fracture?

Answer
- Lack of evidence that early repair (<48 hours) has better outcomes

- Validity of the Bernstine criteria for surgery timings has been questioned (Bernstine et al., Dubois et al.)
- The only two prospective studies on repair timings did not use plates for reconstruction (Dubois et al.)
- Advantages and disadvantages of early surgery (see Case 6.10)
- Indications for early surgery (Box A)

8.4 Question

Examination demonstrates restriction in upwards gaze. How would you manage the patient further and why?

Answer

- Orthoptics assessment: helps ascertain if cause is mechanical restriction, myogenic or neurogenic (Box B)

8.5 Question

Orthoptics assessment demonstrates mild restriction in ocular movements suggestive of entrapment. Would you request a CT scan?

Answer

- Orbital swelling takes approximately six weeks to subside: if diplopia persists at that point then request CT scan

8.6 Question

The patient returns to clinic at 6 weeks having had a CT scan. Can you comment on this CT scan?

Answer

- Sagittal reformat of CT scan showing titanium plate used for orbital floor repair
- Plate is sitting too high posteriorly and does not lie directly on perpendicular plate of palatine bone

8.7 Question

The double vision has now resolved. How would you manage this?

Answer

- Although plate position is sub optimal, clinically the patient is asymptomatic
- No surgery indicated

8.8 Question

On examination you note clinically obvious enophthalmos. What would you do?

Answer

- Clinically obvious enophthalmos is >3–4 mm (see Case 6.10)
- Degree of enophthalmos often difficult to correlate to preoperative defect size on CT

- Counsel patient as to risks of further surgery
- Return to theatre to remove existing plate
- Patient-specific implant (Box C)
- Mirror shape from contralateral orbit

> **Box A: Indications for early repair of orbital fractures (24–48 hours): modified from Burnstine et al.**
>
> - Age: pediatric trapdoor (white-eye)
> - Clinical examination: enophthalmos >2 mm at <48 hours
> - Orthoptics assessment: restriction
> - CT: herniated volume >2 cm^3
> - Early enophthalmos greater than 2 mm
> - Orbital floor +/− medial wall defect >2 cm^2 (likely to result in delayed enophthalmos)

> **Box B. Causes of binocular diplopia**
>
> - Muscular entrapment
> - Neurogenic: injury to cranial nerves III, IV or VI
> - Myogenic: direct injury to muscle, muscle imbalance from altered orbital shape

> **Box C: Areas of difference in orbital fractures**
>
> - Timings: early versus delayed repair
> - Incisions: transconjunctival versus subciliary
> - Repair materials: titanium versus polyethylene or polydioxanone
> - Dissection depth: anatomical landmarks (Box D) versus navigation
> - Plate positioning: intraoperative versus post operative CT
> - Material fabrication: prebent, patient specific
> - Enophthalmos measurements: exophthalmometer versus imaging

> **Box D: Anatomical landmarks and depth measurements**
>
> - Of limited use and require a nondisplaced part of the orbital rim
> - Intraoperative navigation is better but still has limitations
> - Medial wall landmarks (e.g. ethmoidal arteries) unreliable
> - Orbital floor measurements more reliable
> - Inferior orbital rim: inferior orbital fissure (20 mm), apex (40–45 mm)

Further reading

Burnstine MA. Clinical recommendations for repair of isolated orbital floor fractures: An evidence-based analysis. Ophthalmology 2002; 109:1207–1210.

Dubois L, Steenen SA, Gooris PJ, et al. Controversies in orbital reconstruction II. Timing of post-traumatic orbital reconstruction: a systematic review. Int J Oral Maxillofac Surg 2015; 44:433–440.

Gart M, Gosain A. Evidence-based medicine: Orbital floor fractures. Plast Reconstr Surg 2014; 134:1345–1355.

Short case 9: Mandibular condyle fracture

The postoperative patient shown in the figure returns to trauma clinic with the scar.

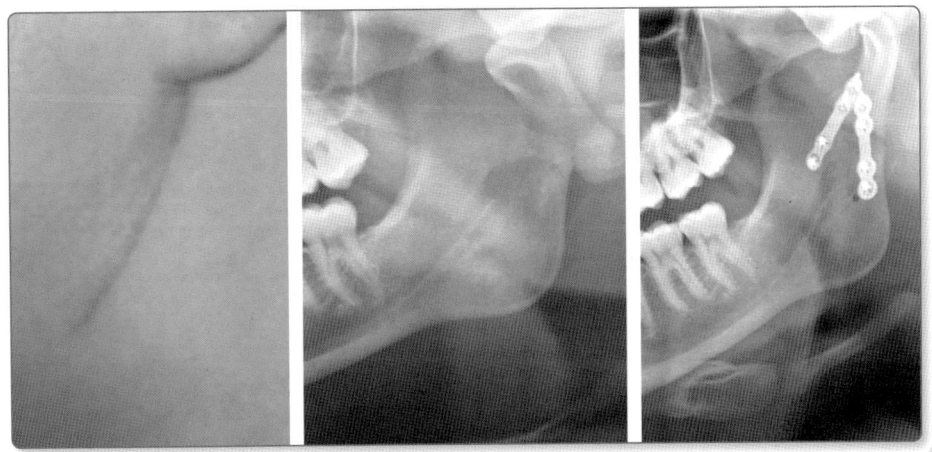

9.1 Question
What are the key points in the history?

Answer

- Retromandibular scar probably represents a transparotid approach to a condyle fracture
- Time since surgery
- Treatment performed
- Other injuries, including other fractures to the mandible
- Occlusion
- General medial health and drug history
- Social history: smoking, diet
- Complications of surgery (Box A)

9.2 Question
How would you examine this patient who is 2 weeks post-surgery?

Answer

Extraoral:
- Scar: healing, other external scars
- Cheek swelling: infection, sialocele
- Mouth opening and deviation
- Facial nerve function

Intraoral:
- Occlusion

9.3 Question

What can you ascertain from the preoperative radiograph?

Answer

- Grossly displaced fracture dislocation of left condylar neck (Box B)
- PA view required to determine whether fragment lies medially or laterally

9.4 Question

Would you request any additional information preoperatively and why?

Answer

- Request a CT if considering surgery (Box C)
- CT will demonstrate any three-dimensional displacement of the condylar head
- CT helps predict ease of reduction and likelihood of significant intraoperative bleeding

9.5 Question

The CT shows that the condyle is dislocated out of the fossa anteriorly and medially. How would you treat them?

Answer

- Such angulation fulfils generally agreed indications for ORIF (Box C)
- Strong evidence that ORIF provides better clinical outcome than closed treatment (Box D)
- Fragment position means unlikely to result in a functioning joint in the long term if MMF alone used

9.6 Question

What are the advantages of ORIF?

Answer

- Improved mouth opening
- Reduced mandibular deviation on opening
- Reduced TMJ pain
- Outcomes superior to closed reduction (Box E)

9.7 Question

Can you comment on this image?

Answer

- ORIF of condylar fracture good reduction
- Two four-hole spaced miniplates using monocortical fixation
- No evidence of MMF
- Need to view the remaining image and second view

9.8 Question

How would you follow-up this patient?

Answer

- No official guidelines on follow-up regime
- Patients undergoing ORIF or closed reduction should have soft diet for 6 weeks
- If MMF was used it should be loosened off or removed completely at 2 weeks
- Mouth opening and guiding exercises required
- After 6 weeks jaw stretching exercises often implemented

Box A: Potential complications of transparotid approach

- Facial nerve weakness: temporary (15%), permanent (1%)
- Scar: hypertrophic (8%)
- Sialocele
- Salivary fistula
- Frey's syndrome
- Malocclusion
- Trismus
- Ankylosis
- Avascular necrosis of the condylar head
- Nonunion

Box B: SORG classification of fracture location

- Utilises the A line, which is taken perpendicular to the posterior border of the mandible through the base of the sigmoid notch
- Condylar neck fracture: >50% fracture above Line A
- Condylar base fracture: >50% fracture below Line A
- Condylar head

Box C: Neff classification of condylar head fractures

Predicts vertical stability of the fracture:
- A: Medial pole only and no loss height
- B: Lateral pole only and potential loss height
- C: Beneath the lateral pole and potential loss height

Box D: Broad indications for ORIF in unilateral condyle fractures

- Zide and Kent: displacement into the middle cranial fossa, lateral extracapsular displacement, failed conservative treatment, open joint
- Joos: shortening of ramus by 4 mm, fragment angulation >37°
- Eckelt: shortening of ramus by 2 mm, fragment angulation >10°

> **Box E: Advantages of closed reduction of condyle fractures**
> - No risks of ORIF, especially facial nerve (Box A)
> - Quicker and technically easier than ORIF
> - Outcomes still generally acceptable to patients

Further reading

Al-Moraissi EA, Ellis E 3rd. Surgical treatment of adult mandibular condylar fractures provides better outcomes than closed treatment: a systematic review and meta-analysis. J Oral Maxillofac Surg 2015; 73:482–493.

Schneider M, Erasmus F, Gerlach KL, et al. Open reduction and internal fixation versus closed treatment and mandibulomaxillary fixation of fractures of the mandibular condylar process: a randomized, prospective, multicenter study with special evaluation of fracture level. J Oral Maxillofac Surg 2008; 66:2537–2544.

Shiju M, Rastogi S, Gupta P, et al. Fractures of the mandibular condyle-Open versus closed-A treatment dilemma. J Craniomaxillofac Surg 2015; 43:448–451.

Short case 10: Zygomaticomaxillary complex fracture

This patient is 10 days after fixation of his zygomaticomaxillary complex (ZMC) fracture.

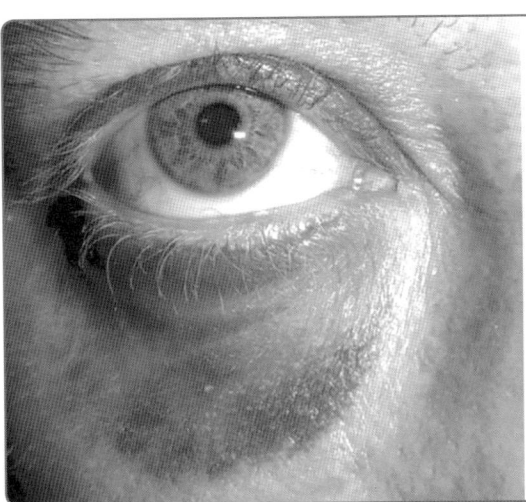
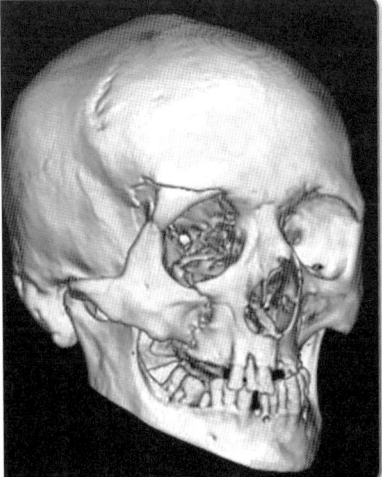

10.1 Question

What are the key points in the history?

Answer

- Mechanism of injury
- Other injuries, especially head and eye injury
- Treatment performed, including surgical approach
- Symptoms prior to and following surgery: numbness, double vision, cheek prominence
- Medical health and drug history
- Social history: occupation (e.g. driver), smoking

10.2 Question

The patient is 10 days after surgery. How would you examine the patient in clinic?

Answer

Extraoral:
- Symmetry and cheek projection
- Numbness
- Facial nerve function
- Eyes: diplopia, restriction in movement, enophthalmos
- Access incisions: transconjunctival, transcutaneous, upper blepharoplasty, coronal flap

Intraoral:
- Occlusion
- Access incision to buttress

10.3 Question

The patient has slight restriction of upward gaze with double vision. How would you manage this?

Answer
- Formal orthoptic and ophthalmology assessment: evidence of mechanical restriction
- No intervention required at this stage
- If no improvement at 6 weeks postoperatively reassess with new CT scan

10.4 Question

What can you ascertain from this patient's preoperative imaging?

Answer
- Three dimensionally reformatted CT scan
- Right ZMC fracture
- Supraorbital fracture potentially involving the frontal sinus
- Unable to clearly see buttress and orbital floor
- Infraorbital rim fractured and displaced
- FZ suture fractured and displaced
- Want to see individual slices to exclude fracture of posterior wall of frontal sinus and potential intracranial injury

10.5 Question

How would you have treated this patient at first presentation?

Answer
- Coronal flap to access and reduce supra orbital fracture
- Neurosurgical input as reduction could result in meningeal tear and CSF leak
- Access and reduce buttress with intraoral vestibular incision
- Access and reduce infraorbital rim with transconjunctival incision
- Repair orbital wall fracture if required
- Utilise navigation and intraoperative CT if available

10.6 Question

What are the potential risks for this patient?

Answer
- Immediate: bleeding necessitating return to theatre
- Early: CSF leak (if intracranial involvement), blindness, diplopia, infection
- Late: asymmetry, numbness, malocclusion, limited mouth opening, enophthalmos, entropion

10.7 Question

Would you repair the orbit at the same time?

Answer

- Decisions are made based upon pre- and intra-operative signs (Box A)
- Arguments exist for and against (Box B)
- In this case orbital floor repair is warranted as patient has restriction and rim already requires fixation (Box C)

10.8 Question

At the 6-week review appointment the patient is still complaining of flattening of their cheek. What would you do?

Answer

- Further treatment should be delayed for 4–6 months
- CT scan
- Unless poor fracture reduction at initial surgery, elective zygomatic osteotomy is unlikely to be helpful
- Cheek can be augmented with autogenous fat or alloplastic material (Medpor or PEEK)

Box A: Decision making to repair orbital walls at same time in ZMC fractures

Preoperative:
- Clinical examination: enophthalmos, hypoglobus
- Orthoptics assessment: restriction
- CT: herniated volume >2 cm^3
- CT: 20% of total orbital volume correlates with enophthamos of 3.5 mm
- CT: orbital floor defect area >50%
- CT: displacement of ZMC complex greater than 10 mm

Intraoperative:
- If orbital rim being accessed for fixation
- Defect size on limited exploration
- Restriction on forced duction test

Box B: Immediate versus delayed orbital repair with ZMC fractures

Argument for immediate repair:
- No second general anaesthetic
- No additional scarring
- Additional risk of damage to eye

Argument for delayed repair:
- May not develop diplopia or altered globe position
- Can use a patient specific implant
- Useful for complex fractures of the orbital frame

> **Box C: Options for management of a flattened cheek following reduction of ZMC fractures**
>
> - Acute return to theatre for reosteotomy: may not be able to osteotomise, risk of unwanted fracture pattern
> - Delayed return to theatre for planned osteotomy: technically more challenging, requires coronal flap and osteotomy at all fracture sites
> - Cheek augmentation with patient specific implant: risk of infection, may need revision as patient ages

Further reading

Choi J, Park SW, Kim J, et al. Predicting late enophthalmos: Differences between medial and inferior orbital wall fractures. J Plast Reconstr Aesthet Surg 2016; 69:e238–e244.

Carls F, Schuknecht B, Sailer HF. Orbital volumetry as a planning principle for reconstruction of the orbital wall. Fortschr Kiefer Gesichtschir 1994; 39:23–27.

Tahernia A, Erdmann D, Follmar K, et al. Clinical implications of orbital volume change in the management of isolated and zygomaticomaxillary complex-associated orbital floor injuries. Plast Reconstr Surg 2009; 123:968–975.

Long case 11: Panfacial fractures

This patient shown in the figure was involved in a car accident 6 weeks ago.

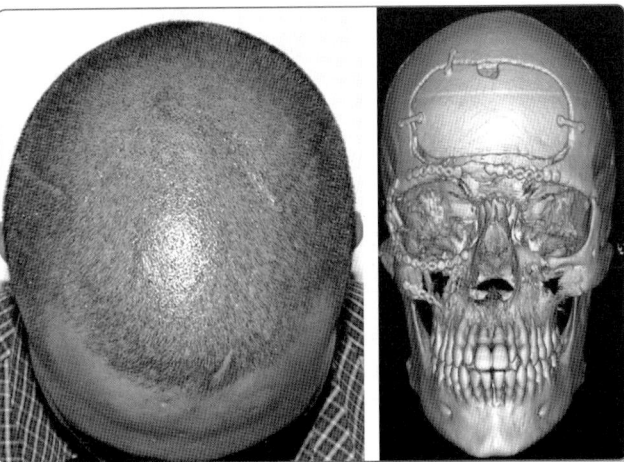

1. **Scenario**

   Assess the patient and provide a proposed management plan

2. **Preparation**
   - Use the time to introduce yourself, clean your hands and obtain consent to assess
   - Position the patient and try to provide a spot diagnosis

3. **History**
   - Stay calm, build rapport and try not to miss key points, e.g. the social history
   - Do not rush straight into an examination
   - Identify a reason for surgery and any potential complications

4. **Examination**
   - Assess from front, above, side and below
   - Use exophthalmometer if present
   - Ascertain projection, weakness, numbness, incisions, occlusion
   - Work either top to bottom, or bottom to top
   - Ensure all main buttresses are palpated
   - A full cranial nerve evaluation should be performed

5. **Investigation**
   - Imaging: OPG, CT
   - Photographs
   - Three-dimensional printed model

6. **Summarise**
    - Thank the patient and then turn directly to the examiner and summarise your findings

7. **Treatment plan**
    - Surgical objectives
    - Focus on a clear plan (short and long term)
    - Remember there is rarely one correct answer
    - Emphasise the need for multidisciplinary management

Box A: Concept of the trauma long case

- A 15-minute assessment likely encompassing the structure above
- Follow-up trauma patients in clinic are common, but often poor attenders to examinations
- Preoperative patients may be present on the ward prior to surgery
- A long case will usually be either a panfacial, nasoethmoidal, or frontal sinus fractures or some combination

---

Box B: Arguments to get clear in your head regarding panfacial fractures

- One or two stages (e.g. mandible plus tracheostomy as stage one)
- Sequencing
- Should orbital floor fractures be repaired concurrently?
- Airway options: pros and cons of tracheotomy, submental intubation, regular intubation

---

Box C: Arguments for two-stage operating

- Conforms to the concept of reduced length surgical procedure, i.e. Damage control surgery
- A surgical airway enables the patient to be weaned off sedation
- This in turn enables assessment of neurological function (prognosis) and eye movements (need for orbital wall repair)
- Getting the transverse width of the mandible correct first greatly aids with reduction of the mid face in the transverse dimension

---

Box D: Little tips in panfacial fractures

- The correct sequence is the one that begins with fixing the bones to those you feel most confident are in the correct place
- Waiting to perform surgery may reduce swelling but it makes reduction more difficult
- The zygomatic arch may be used to get the AP distance but it is easy to make it too bowed as the arch actually straight
- Consider performing the lower eyelid incisions first due to oedema produced by the coronal flap
- Orbital floors are usually repaired at very end when you are most tired

Further reading

Kelly K, Manson PN, Vander Kolk CA, et al. Sequencing LeFort fracture treatment (Organization of treatment for a panfacial fracture). J Craniofac Surg 1990; 1:168–178.

Markowitz BL, Manson PN. Panfacial fractures: organization of treatment. Clin Plast Surg 1989; 16:105–114.

Chapter 6
Salivary gland disease

SHORT CASES

1. Recurrent submandibular gland swelling from a sialolith
2. Rapidly growing submandibular gland lump
3. Slow growing parotid gland lump
4. Post submandibular gland excision
5. Post parotid gland excision
6. Ranula in the floor of mouth

LONG CASE

7. Superficial parotidectomy following recurrent sialadenitis

Short case 1: Recurrent submandibular gland swelling from a sialolith

The patient shown in the figure has been referred in for recurrent submandibular swelling.

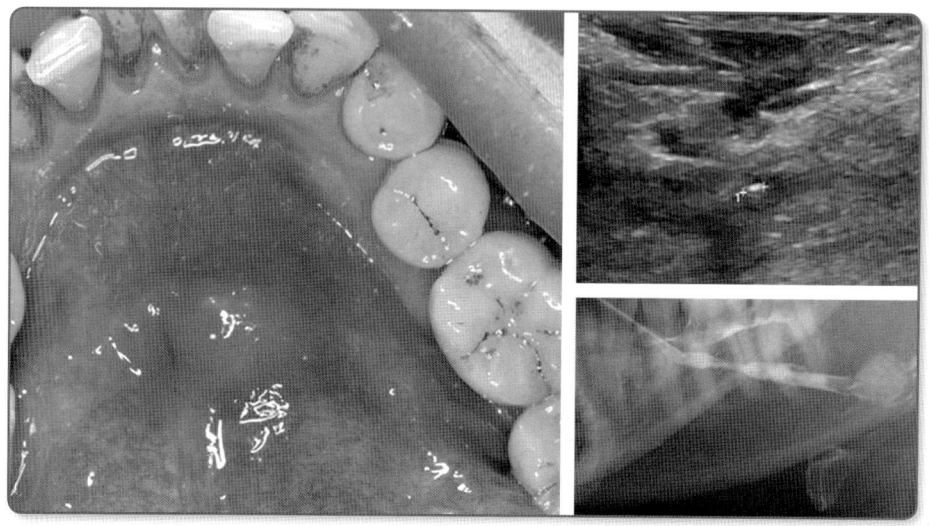

1.1 Question
What are the pertinent points in the history?

Answer

- Differentiate between submandibular gland and lymph node swelling
- Submandibular: mealtime syndrome, previous stones, dehydration, autoimmune diseases
- Lymph node: other swollen nodes, general causes of lymphadenopathy
- Past medical, drug and social history

1.2 Question
What are the key points in the examination?

Answer

- Inspection: submandibular swelling, duct orifice (inflammation, pus)
- Bimanual palpation: submandibular gland, floor of mouth for stone
- Attempt to express saliva from duct
- Cervical lymph nodes

1.3 Question
Examination demonstrates an isolated tender enlarged submandibular gland. How would you investigate this further?

Short case 1 Recurrent submandibular gland swelling from a sialolith

Answer
- OPG: stones (Box A), dental pathology causing lymphadenopathy
- Ultrasound

1.4 Question
What can ultrasound tell you?

Answer
- Nature: gland, node, separate mass (e.g. tumour)
- Duct: dilatation, strictures
- Glandular features: sialectasis
- Stones: size (>3 mm), location (gland, hilum, and distal duct)

1.5 Question
Ultrasound identifies an enlarged, hypoechoic submandibular gland with a dilated duct but no other pathology. What would be your next course of action?

Answer
- Recurrent swelling and a dilated duct suggest benign obstructive pathology
- A sialogram should be deferred if the gland is tender as this suggests potential active infection
- Most clinicians would suggest MRI over CT scan

1.6 Question
The MRI demonstrates an enlarged, inflamed gland but no other pathology. How would you manage the patient?

Answer
- No one correct answer for this!
- Manage symptoms conservatively: antibiotics if required
- Sialogram after 6 weeks

1.7 Question
The sialogram demonstrates a small 3 mm stone, just distal to the hilum. How would you manage this?

Answer
- Conservative
- Sialography and retrieval (Box B)
- Sialendoscopy and retrieval (Box C)
- Lithotripsy (Box D)
- Surgical stone excision (Box E)
- Gland excision

Box A: Sialolithiasis

- Incidence: submandibular (90%), parotid (10%), minor (1%)
- Radiopacity: submandibular (80%), parotid (60%)
- Contributory factors: dehydration, sepsis, stricture

Box B: Basket retrieval of stones

- Can be performed using sialography or endoscopy
- Only suitable for small stones (3–5 mm, or <30% larger than the duct diameter)
- Ideally stone is mobile
- No stricture in front of the stone

Box C: Sialendoscopy

- Flexible endoscope passed down the duct
- Local anaesthetic used around the papilla
- Direct view of causes of duct obstruction
- Can remove calculi or dilate strictures
- Cannot see intraparenchymal calculi
- Operator dependent

Box D: Shockwave lithotripsy

- Generally performed by extracorporeal method
- Suitable for stones about 5–8 mm in diameter
- Limited locations perform it
- Multiple attendances required
- Published results are a 60% stone clearance

Box E: Surgical removal of calculi

- Usually performed for large stones or ones close to the papilla
- Complications: infection, lingual nerve damage, stricture, stone recurrence

Further reading

Carta F, Farneti P, Cantore S, et al. Sialendoscopy for salivary stones: principles, technical skills and therapeutic experience. Acta Otorhinolaryngol Ital 2017; 37:102–112.

Desmots F, Chossegros C, Salles F, et al. Lithotripsy for salivary stones with prospective US assessment on our first 25 consecutive patients. J Craniomaxillofac Surg 2014; 42:577–582.

Short case 2: Rapidly growing submandibular gland lump

The patient in this figure has attended your rapid access neck lump clinic with a slowly growing lump over the angle of her mandible.

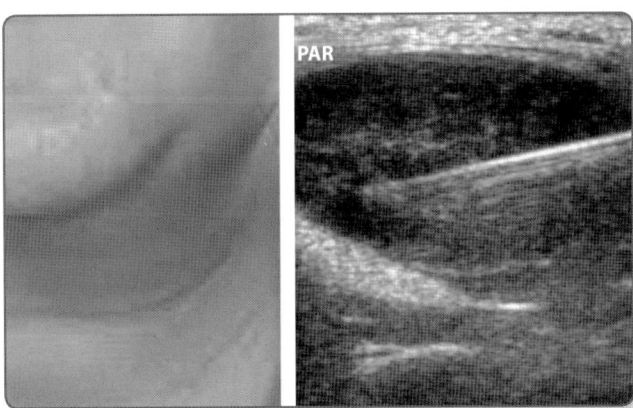

2.1 Question

How would you assess the pertinent history?

Answer

- Discrete lump (Box A) or diffuse enlargement (Box B)
- Fluctuating in size (usually benign or lymph node), or continually growing
- Speed of growth (benign/malignant)
- Pain: constant, associated with meals (mealtime syndrome)
- Red flags: B type symptoms (Box C)
- Past medical, drug and social history

2.2 Question

This is a rapidly growing lump. What are the key points in the examination?

Answer

- End of bed: general health, obvious lump or scar
- Inspection: size, overlying skin changes
- Bimanual palpation: discrete lump or enlargement of the whole gland
- Test nerves: marginal mandibular, hypoglossal, lingual
- Intraoral: other causes of lumps (oral SCC, dental infection), express saliva from duct
- Cervical lymphadenopathy

2.3 Question

This is a single discrete submandibular lump. How would you investigate this?

Answer

- Ultrasound-guided FNA
- Core biopsy

2.4 Question

Ultrasound demonstrates a mass within the submandibular gland but the FNA is nondiagnostic. How would you manage the patient?

Answer

- Strong suggestion of a submandibular gland tumour
- Need to ascertain if benign or malignant as this determines surgery
- Repeat ultrasound-guided FNA or core biopsy
- Many clinicians would request an MRI head and neck due to rapid growth

2.5 Question

Would you request a CT or MRI?

Answer

- MRI remains superior to CT in tumour structure analysis should this be suspected
- CT should be reserved for cases when MRI contraindicated, e.g. pacemaker, metallic foreign bodies

2.6 Question

What are the potential advantages of core biopsy over FNA?

Answer

- Preserves tissue architecture
- Enables diagnosis of lymphoma
- Has a greater sensitivity in diagnosing benign versus malignant (97% versus 80–90% for FNAC)
- More likely to make the correct histological diagnosis (87% versus 70% for ultrasound)

2.7 Question

Why do many hospital departments then not offer core biopsy?

Answer

- Expensive and time consuming
- Greater risk of complications such as bleeding
- Risk of tumour seeding (highly controversial)

2.8 Question

The patient in the figure has repeat FNA which demonstrates no evidence of atypia but cannot suggest a diagnosis. The MRI demonstrates a mass but nothing else. How would you manage this?

Answer
- All investigations suggest a benign neoplasm
- Excision of submandibular gland is warranted

Box A: Causes of discrete lumps within salivary glands

- Salivary cysts
- Benign epithelial tumours
- Malignant epithelial tumours
- Metastatic SCC
- Benign connective tissue tumours
- Sarcomas
- Lymphomas
- Chronic sclerosing sialadenitis
- Adenomatoid hyperplasia
- Oncocytosis

Box B: Causes of diffuse gland enlargement

- Sialadenitis
- Sialosis
- Sjögren's syndrome
- Mikulicz's disease and syndrome
- Sarcoidois
- MALToma: only cancer that produces a diffuse swelling

Box C: 'B-type' symptoms suggestive of non-Hodgkins lymphoma

- Fever
- Lymphadenopathy: neck, underarms, groin
- Night sweats and/or chills
- Fatigue
- Loss of appetite, nausea, vomiting
- Unexplained weight loss

Further reading

Novoa E, Gurtler N, Arnoux A, Kraft M. Role of ultrasound-guided core-needle biopsy in the assessment of head and neck lesions: a meta-analysis and systematic review of the literature. Head Neck 2012; 34:1497–1503.

Schmidt RL, Hall BJ, Wilson AR, et al. A systematic review and meta-analysis of the diagnostic accuracy of fine-needle aspiration cytology for parotid gland lesions. Am J Clin Pathol 2011; 136:45–59.

Short case 3: Slow growing parotid gland lump

The patient shown in the figure has attended your rapid access neck lump clinic with a slowly growing lump over the angle of her mandible.

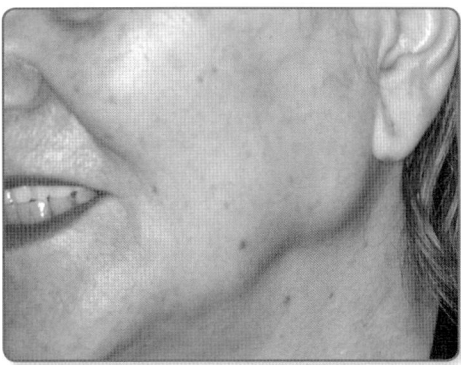

3.1 Question
What are the key points in the examination?

Answer
- Inspect gland: skin erythema or ulceration, scars from previous surgery
- Inspect ear and scalp: for a potential primary: usually SCC or melanoma
- Palpate gland bimanually: location, discrete lump or enlargement of the whole gland
- Palpate for cervical lymphadenopathy
- Facial nerve: assess all branches for weakness
- Intraoral: other causes of lumps (oral SCC, dental infection), express saliva from parotid duct
- Flexible nasendoscopy: parapharyngeal extension

3.2 Question
How will ultrasound help you?

Answer
- WIll indicate if lesion is within gland, whether it is cystic or solid, and can detect local metastases (Box A)
- In some cases, may be able to suggest malignancy, or not

3.3 Question
Ultrasound-guided FNA demonstrates a small well circumscribed mass but some atypical features. How would you manage the patient?

Answer
- Ultrasound (Box A)

- MRI: required to assess large or poorly defined lesions, or those showing atypical features on USS. Often requested even for a benign presentation (Box B)

3.4 Question

MRI confirms a 2-cm lesion confined to the superficial lobe. FNA suggests pleomorphic adenoma (PA) in the parotid tail. How would you treat the patient?

Answer
- Superficial parotidectomy or extracapsular dissection

3.5 Question

The patient underwent superficial parotidectomy but histology is suggestive of low-grade acinic cell carcinoma. How would you manage the patient?

Answer
- Review histology: completeness of excision, extraparenchymal extension
- Imaging of neck and chest: for staging (Box B)

3.6 Question

The mass was 2 cm in diameter, and there is no evidence of regional or distant metastasis. How would you stage the patient?

Answer
- Staging of salivary gland malignancy is the same as oral cancer except for the primary lesion (Box C)
- This patient is group stage 1 (T1, N0, M0)

3.7 Question

Does the patient need radiotherapy?

Answer
- No indication for radiotherapy (Box D)

Box A: Role of ultrasound

Advantages
- Can tell if intra- or extraglandular
- Can tell if cystic or solid
- Can detect nodal metastases

Disadvantages
- Cannot see deep lobe of parotid
- Cannot assess perineural spread
- Cannot gain much information from screenshots when looked at later
- Operator dependent

Box B: Role of MRI in salivary gland assessment

- Detect if deep lobe involvement (USS can't do this)
- Detect perineural invasion (USS can't do this)
- Define if gland or node within gland
- Assess extraparenchymal extension (EPE) and invasion (e.g. parapharyngeal space)
- Detect nodal metastasis
- Movement artefact as slow acquisition time, pacemakers, metallic objects, claustrophobic

Box C: Tumour (T) staging of salivary gland malignancy

- TX: Primary tumour cannot be assessed
- T0: No tumour present
- Tis: Carcinoma in situ
- T1: Tumour ≤2 cm (no extraparenchymal extension)
- T2: Tumour 2–4 cm (no extraparenchymal extension)
- T3: Tumour >4 cm and/or extraparenchymal extension (no 7th nerve involvement)
- T4a: Tumour invades skin, mandible, ear canal, and/or facial nerve
- T4b: Tumour invades skull base, pterygoid plates, and/or carotid artery

Box D: Indications for adjuvant radiotherapy

- Incomplete margins
- High grade tumour
- Perineural invasion: field should go up to base of skull
- Tumour spillage
- Lymph node metastases
- Enucleation of the tumour
- Extraparotid extension
- T3 and T4 (i.e. >4 cm, the '4 cm rule')
- Recurrent PSA

Further reading

Sood S, McGurk M, Vaz F, et al. Management of Salivary Gland Tumours: United Kingdom National Multidisciplinary Guidelines. J Laryngol Otol 2016; 130:S142–S149.

Short case 4: Post submandibular gland excision

This patient had elective surgery to neck a few weeks ago.

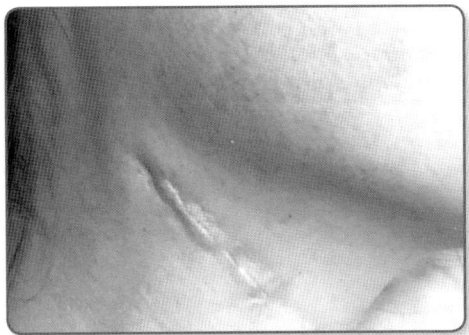

4.1 Question
How would you assess the patient?

Answer

- Inspect: incision for location (submandibular), infection, abnormal healing such as hypertrophy
- Inspect: duct orifice for erythema, stone
- Inspect marginal mandibular nerve function: lower lip weakness
- Inspect: hypoglossal nerve function (protrude tongue)
- Palpate: floor of mouth bimanually
- Palpate: cervical lymphadenopathy
- Palpate: lingual nerve function (sensation)

4.2 Question
Preoperative assessment was highly suggestive of malignancy. How would you manage this?

Answer

- FNA or code biopsy result: high or low grade
- Stage the patient: MRI head and neck, CT chest
- Discuss at the head and neck MDT
- Take into account patient's wishes, medical history and social circumstances

4.3 Question
Imaging identifies a 3-cm lesion without local or regional metastasis. What surgical treatment would you recommend?

Answer
- Level 1 neck dissection only (Box B)

4.4 Question

The histology comes back as 1 cm high grade adenocarcinoma with no local or distant metastasis. How would you manage this?

Answer
- Discuss at head and neck MDT
- High-grade lesions require selective neck dissection of levels 1–3 (Box B)
- Radiotherapy recommended for adenoid cystic carcinoma (see scenario 7.3)

4.5 Question

Would you give chemotherapy?

Answer
- No indication for chemotherapy (Box C)

4.6 Question

How would you follow patient up?

Answer
- Review the patient every 6–8 weeks for 2 years
- Limited evidence exists to support the type and frequency of follow-up imaging
- Ultrasound is often requested every 3 months but is unhelpful for visualising deep compartments

---

Box A: Treatment of submandibular gland if carcinoma suggested preoperatively

- Extracapsular dissection of the gland
- Treat high-grade lesions aggressively with an additional 2 cm of healthy tissue
- Sacrifice of nerve if within resection margin
- Bone involvement requires resection

Box B: Treatment of neck in known salivary gland carcinoma

- Currently based upon poor evidence
- N0 (low grade tumour): level 1 neck dissection
- N0 (high grade): selective 2–4 (parotid), selective 1–3 (submandibular)
- N1: selective 1–4

> **Box C: Indications for chemotherapy in biopsy proven salivary gland carcinoma**
> - Used for distant metastases only
> - Current agents not very effective for metastatic salivary gland disease
> - Cisplatin is the most commonly used agent
> - Biological agents such as Cetuximab have been used

Further reading

Freling N, Crippa F, Maroldi R. Staging and follow-up of high-grade malignant salivary gland tumours: The role of traditional versus functional imaging approaches – A review. Oral Oncol 2016; 60:157–166.

Short case 5: Post parotid gland excision

The patient shown in the figure returns to clinic following surgery.

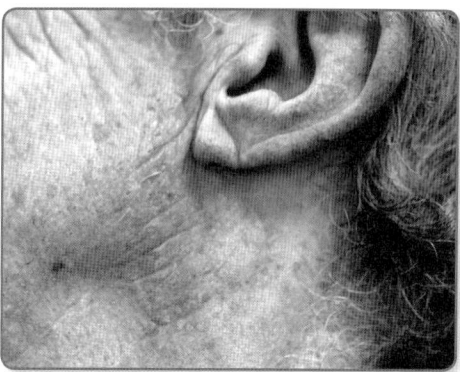

5.1 Question
What can you see in the figure?

Answer
- Scar from a left modified Blair preauricular incision with a submandibular extension (consistent with surgery to the parotid gland)

5.2 Question
How would you assess the patient?

Answer
- History: reason for surgery, postoperative complications (Box A), preoperative facial nerve function
- Operation note: type of operation (Box B), tumour spillage
- Examination: scar, facial nerve, greater auricular nerve
- Ultrasound-guided FNA

5.3 Question
Preoperative assessment was highly suggestive of malignancy. How would you manage this?

Answer
- Stage the patient: MRI head and neck, CT chest
- Discuss at head and neck MDT
- Take into account patient's wishes, medical history and social circumstances

5.4 Question
Preoperative imaging identified a 2-cm lesion in the superficial lobe without local or regional metastasis. What treatment would you recommended?

Answer

- Total conservative parotidectomy is default position for malignancy (Box C)
- No indication for neck dissection

5.5 Question

Intraoperatively the lesion is enveloping the facial nerve. Would you sacrifice the nerve?

Answer

- Always attempt to preserve nerve if functioning preoperatively, even if mass is closely associated with it
- Only sacrifice nerve if completely enveloped by tumour and unable to separate from mass (Box D)
- Rely on radiotherapy to destroy micrometastasis
- Intraoperative nerve sacrifice should be repaired with interpositional nerve graft

5.6 Question

What would you like to know in the histology results to determine any further treatment?

Answer

- Tumour type
- Size
- Completeness of excision
- Intraoperative spillage
- Tumour grade
- Perineural invasion

5.7 Question

Histology comes back as a fully excised 3 cm high-grade adenoid cystic carcinoma. What further treatment would you recommend?

Answer

- Radiotherapy should be given for adenoid cystic carcinomas, due to close proximity of nerve to tumour
- No indication for chemotherapy

Box A: Complications of parotidectomy

- Immediate: button hole flap, tumour spillage, facial and greater auricular nerve injury, haematoma
- Early: wound breakdown, infection
- Late: scar, retromandibular deformity, Freys syndrome, sialocele

> **Box B: Parotidectomy classification**
>
> Nerve dissection:
> - Partial superficial parotidectomy: dissect only those going into tumour. Only part of superficial gland excised
> - Superficial parotidectomy: dissect all 5 branches. All of superficial part of gland excised
> - Total conservative parotidectomy: excise all parotid tissue superficial and deep to the nerve with nerve preservation
> - Radical total parotidectomy – as above but sacrifice of nerve
> - Selective deep lobe parotidectomy – superficial lobe remains pedicled
>
> No nerve dissection:
> - Extracapsular dissection: preauricular flap, tumour removed in extracapsular plane with small cuff of surrounding tissue. Nerve only dissected if runs into field
> - Enucleation: incision over lump, capsule opened, contents removed and capsule left in situ. Never used anymore

> **Box C: Management of parotid malignancy**
>
> - Total conservative parotidectomy: default position for malignancy [McGurk book]
> - Superficial parotidectomy: increasingly advocated for young patients with small, low-grade tumours in the parotid tail

> **Box D: Indications for facial nerve sacrifice**
>
> - Preoperative paralysis
> - Recurrent malignancy
> - Gross encasement and infiltration of gland

Further reading

McGurk M, Combes J. Controversies in the Management of Salivary Gland Disease, 2nd Edition. Oxford University Press, 2011.

Short case 6: Ranula in the floor of mouth

This 20-year-old patient complains of an intermittent swelling in the floor of their mouth.

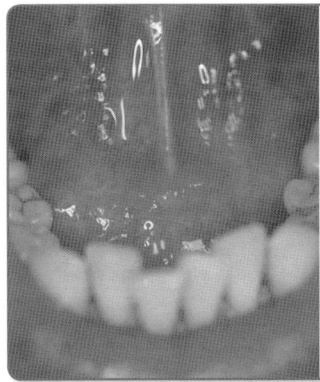
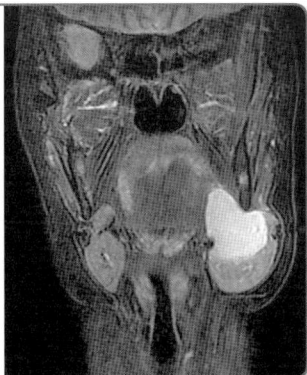

6.1 Question

What is your differential diagnosis?

Answer

- Ranula (Box A)
- Vascular malformation
- Lymphadenitis
- Dermoid cyst

6.2 Question

How would you assess the patient in clinic?

Answer

- Assessment comprises: tailored history, consent for examination and requesting pertinent imaging

6.3 Question

What are the key points in the history?

Answer

- Present since birth (congenital) or post traumatic (acquired)
- Bleeding: vascular malformation
- Neck swelling: plunging ranula
- Exacerbations with upper respiratory tract infections (lymphadenitis, lymphatic malformation)

6.4 Question

What are the key points in the examination?

Answer

- Intraoral: size, colour, airway compromise
- Extraoral: swelling

6.5 Question

What investigations would you request and why?

Answer

- Doppler ultrasound: assess size, extension into the neck, vascularity
- MRI: fully assess extent

6.6 Question

The patient had the MRI. What can you see?

Answer

- Short tau inversion-recovery (STIR) sequence MRI in coronal section
- Well circumscribed high signal intensity lesion in the floor the mouth herniating through mylohyoid muscle
- consistent with a plunging ranula (Box B)

6.7 Question

How would you treat an intraoral ranula that is not plunging?

Answer

- Conservative: if small and not causing problems
- Excision of sublingual gland: the best surgical option
- Marsupialisation: by deroofing is not usually successful
- Ablation of cyst lining: laser, sclerotherapy – both aim to produce scar tissue that obstructs duct
- Removal of ranula alone is not usually successful

6.8 Question

How would you treat a plunging ranula?

Answer

- Intraoral approach
- Follow ranula through mylohyoid to find its base
- Remove sublingual gland

Box A: Definition of a ranula

- A ranula occurs when a salivary gland unit within the sublingual gland ejects saliva beneath the mucosa causing an extravasation cyst
- A plunging ranula occurs when the cyst extends below the mylohyoid muscle

Box B: Appearance of a ranula on imaging

- Well defined, unilocular lesion situated off the midline in the sublingual space, superficial to mylohyoid and related to the sublingual gland
- Ultrasound: anechoic cystic structure
- MRI: high signal intensity lesion in T2 weighted images

Further reading

Dias FL, Lima RA, Cernea CR. Management of Tumors of the Submandibular and Sublingual Glands. Chapter 21. In: Myers E, Salivary gland disorders, 1st Edition. Springer 2007.

Long case 7: Superficial parotidectomy following recurrent sialadenitis

This patient is 10-day postsurgery.

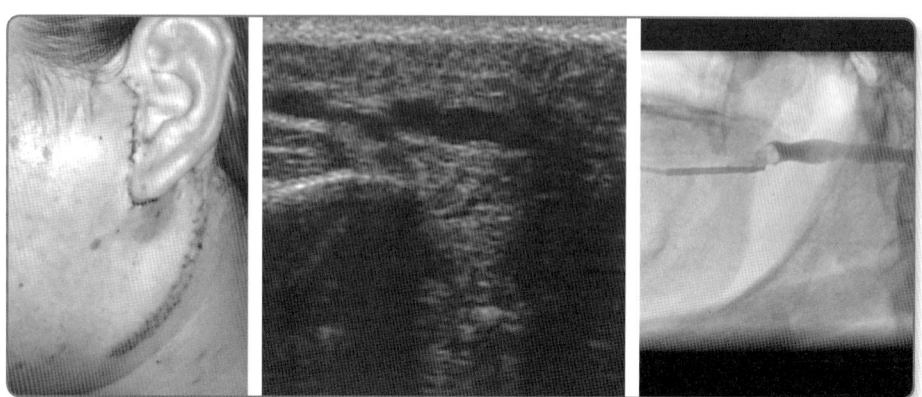

7.1 Question
How would you assess the patient shown in this figure as a long clinical case?

Answer
- This patient has a recently closed incision for surgery to treat parotid gland pathology (Box A)
- A large number of reasons for this type of surgery exist and include non-salivary gland causes (e.g. TMJ pathology or condylar trauma)
- Full assessment would comprise the steps shown in Box B

7.2 Question
What are the key points in the history?

Answer
- Identify reason for surgery
- Risk factors for sialadenitis (Box C)
- Postoperative complaints: weakness, numbness, swelling, pain, bleeding
- History of original complaint: recurrent infections, response to antibiotics
- Previous treatment: surgical, radiological, endoscopic
- Past medical history including allergies
- Drug history: anticoagulation, immunosuppression
- Social history: postoperative support, relationships

Long case 7 Superficial parotidectomy following recurrent sialadenitis

7.3 Question
What are the key points in the examination?

Answer
- Wound site: incision type (in this case modified Blair), erythema
- Surrounding area: swelling, sialocele, Frey's syndrome
- Facial nerve function (Box D)
- Earlobe numbness
- Intraoral: parotid duct orifice

7.4 Question
What investigations would you request and why?

Answer
- Sialogram: identifies likely cause for surgery (in this case a sialolith)
- Ultrasound: most likely a report (this scan shows duct dilatation)
- Cytology or core biopsy result: for an oncology case
- CT or MRI

7.5 Question
How would you summarise appropriately?

Answer
- Thank the patient and ask if there is anything pertinent you have missed?
- Turn to the examiner and summarise
- Classification of parotidectomy: in this scenario total conservative parotidectomy
- Emphasise the need for multidisciplinary management

7.6 Question
What are the alternative treatment options for recurrent sialadenitis?

Answer
- Radiological guided and endoscopic techniques
- Aspiration of sialocele, management of Frey's

Box A: Concept of a salivary long case
- A 15-minute assessment likely encompassing the structure above
- Other potential scenarios include pre- and postoperative submandibular or parotid gland lumps, obstructive and neoplastic cases
- Concepts include the need for MRI, risks to the facial nerve of different types of surgery and indications for neck dissections and radiotherapy

> **Box B: Structuring a salivary gland long case assessment**
> - Introduction and consent to assess
> - Patient positioning while cleaning hands
> - Tailored history
> - Examination
> - Review of any available investigations
> - Summary back to the patient
> - Differential diagnosis

> **Box C: Risk factors for sialadenitis**
> - Obstruction: stone, stricture
> - Infective: bacterial, viral
> - Granulomatous disease: tuberculosis, sarcoidosis
> - Sjögren's disease
> - Immunosuppression including diabetes
> - Dehydration

> **Box D: Risks of facial nerve injury following parotidectomy for sialadenitis**
> - Superficial parotidectomy: 30% (temporary), 1–3% (permanent)
> - Total parotidectomy: 50% (temporary), 1–3% (permanent)

Further reading

Patel R, Low T, Gao K, O'Brien C. Clinical outcome after surgery for 75 patients with parotid sialadenitis. Laryngoscope 2007; 117:644–647.

Chapter 7

Oral pathology

SHORT CASES

1. Medication-related osteonecrosis of the jaw (MRONJ)
2. Necrotising sialometaplasia and oral ulcers
3. Fibrous dysplasia
4. mucous membrane pemphigoid
5. Oral lichen planus
6. Oral pigmentation and mucosal melanoma
7. Oral white patch and premalignancy
8. Osteoradionecrosis in the mandible
9. Gingival mass
10. Keratocystic odontogenic tumour
11. Calcifying epithelial odontogenic tumour

LONG CASE

12. Recurrent multicystic ameloblastoma

Short case 1: Medication-related osteonecrosis of the jaw (MRONJ)

The patient shown in the figure recently had a tooth extracted by their dentist and is noting a foul taste in their mouth.

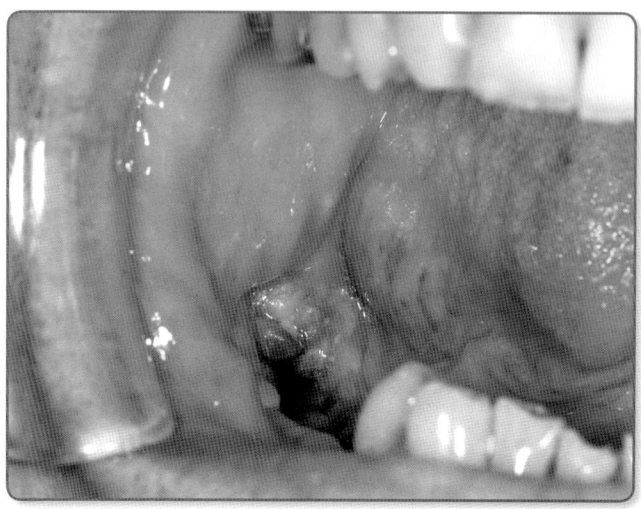

1.1 Question

What can you see in the figure and what is the likely diagnosis?

Answer

- This patient has exposed bone in left mandible presumably where tooth was extracted
- Likely diagnosis is either MRONJ or osteoradionecrosis (ORN)
- Exclude neoplasia (Box A)

1.2 Question

What are the key points in the history?

Answer

- Presenting complaint: pain, dietary intake
- Medical history: cancer, osteoporosis, radiotherapy
- Drug history: anti-resorptive and antiangiogenic drugs

1.3 Question

This patient has been on zolendronate infusions for the spinal deposits of his prostate cancer. What are the key points in the examination?

Answer

- Extraoral: lymphadenopathy, cutaneous sinus
- Intraoral: mucosal dehiscence, lip or tongue numbness, pathological fracture

Short case 1 Medication-related osteonecrosis of the jaw (MRONJ)

1.4 Question
What investigations would you perform?

Answer

- OPG: size of necrotic area, relationship to inferior alveolar nerve and tooth root tips, pathological fracture
- CT: size of necrotic area, lymphadenopathy
- Biopsy: to exclude neoplasia
- C-terminal cross-linking telopeptide (CTX) test (Box A)

1.5 Question
How would you stage this asymptomatic patient?

Answer

- Using the AAOMS 2014 staging (this patient is stage I)

1.6 Question
How would you manage stage I disease?

Answer

- Good oral hygiene, chlorhexidine mouthwashes and oral antibiotics for flare ups (co-amoxiclav or doxycycline)

1.7 Question
The patient's dentist has asked for the retained lower third molar tooth to be extracted so they can make a denture. How would you proceed?

Answer

- No correct answer for this so be certain in your choice!
- Assess whether patient can manage without a denture
- If they insist upon a denture consider extraction of the tooth first
- Attempt to quieten the disease with oral antibiotics prior to the surgery
- Some clinicians advocate hyperbaric oxygen treatment prior to extraction in high-risk patients

1.8 Question
The dentist asks you to extract a tooth on the contralateral nonaffected side. What would you advise?

Answer

- All attempts should be made to conserve teeth rather than extract
- Patients should be stratified into low risk and high risk. Low-risk patients (oral bisphosphonates) can have extractions in a dental practice using an atraumatic technique
- High-risk patients (intravenous bisphosphonates) should be treated in hospital

- Chlorhexidine mouthwash should be used for 2 minutes preoperatively and the patient reviewed for healing 2 weeks later
- No evidence for antibiotics but many clinicians still prescribe for 5 days
- Risk of developing MRONJ following oral bisphosponates for osteoporosis is 0.1–0.5% (Box E)

1.9 Question

Would you give the patient a drug holiday first?

Answer

- Drug holiday may be considered for patients who have been on oral bisphosphonates for more than 4 years
- No evidence it reduces the risk of developing MRONJ
- For those clinicians utilising CTX, a drug holiday is quoted as resulting in serum levels increasing approximately 25 units per month, and they wait until the value is above 150
- For oncology patients on current intravenous denosumab infusions consider advising an alternative drug

---

Box A: Differential diagnosis of exposed bone in the alveolus

- Infection: osteitis, osteomyelitis
- Neoplasia: recurrent squamous cell carcinoma (SCC), metastasis
- Iatrogenic: ORN, MRONJ

Box B: The role of CTX in risk stratification for developing MRONJ following extractions in patients taking oral bisphosphonates

- Some studies have reported that a CTX level lower than 150 pg/mL is associated with a greater risk
- Two systematic reviews in 2017 found that CTX has no predictive value in risk stratification
- The 2014 American Association of Oral and Maxillofacial Surgeons (AAOMS) guidelines do not recommend its use due to the lack of supporting data

---

Box C: AAOMS 2014 guidelines for staging

- Stage 0: vague symptoms but no exposed bone
- Stage 1: exposed bone localised to alveolus (i.e. not beyond tooth roots)
- Stage 2: exposed bone that is painful
- Stage 3: necrotic bone past alveolus, cutaneous fistula, fracture

> **Box D: AAOMS 2014 guidelines for treatment**
> - Stage 1: chlorhexidine mouthwash and antibiotics as required
> - Stage 2: consider sequestrotomy and mucosal closure
> - Stage 3: consider resection and a vascularised bone graft

> **Box E: Rule of thumb risks of developing MRONJ following tooth extractions**
>
> Noncancer patients
> - Oral bisphosphonates <4 years: 0.1%
> - Oral bisphosphonates >4 years: 0.2%
>
> Cancer patients
> - IV zolendronate: 1% (but dose dependent)
> - Denosunab: 0.7–2%

Further reading

Dal Prá K. Efficacy of the C-terminal telopeptide test in predicting the development of bisphosphonate-related osteonecrosis of the jaw: a systematic review. Int J Oral Maxillofac Surg 2017; 46:151–156.

Ruggiero S. American Association of Oral and Maxillofacial Surgeons position paper on medication-related osteonecrosis of the jaw-2014 update. J Oral Maxillofac Surg 2014; 72:1938–1956.

Short case 2: Necrotising sialometaplasia and oral ulcers

This patient attends with a slowly growing left cheek mass.

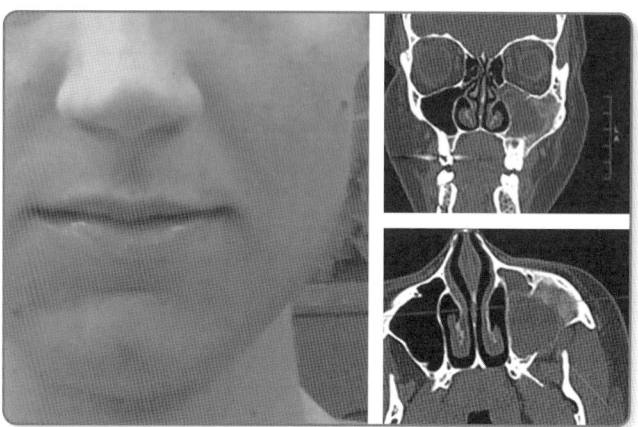

2.1 Question

What can you see in this figure and what is the likely diagnosis?

Answer

- This figure demonstrates an ulcerative lesion in midline of palate and most likely represents necrotising sialometaplasia
- Main differential diagnoses include: neoplasia, Wegener's granulomatosis and lymphoma
- Other causes of oral ulcer shown in Box A

2.2 Question

What are the relevant points in the history?

Answer

- Presenting complaint: previous ulcers, trauma, size, frequency, duration, critical features since self-limiting and extraoral ulceration (ulcers elsewhere in body)
- Past medial history: bowel joint or eye problems
- Drug history: nicorandil
- Social history: smoking, sexual history

2.3 Question

What are the relevant points in the examination?

Answer

- A comprehensive examination for pathological lesions presenting in the oral cavity is shown in Box B
- Pertinent points specifically for assessment of an oral ulcer include:
  - Ulcer: site, size, shape, consistency (Box C)
  - Remaining oral cavity: other ulcers or lesions, scarring from previous lesions
  - Cervical lymph nodes

2.4 Question

How would you explain necrotising sialometaplasia to the patient?

Answer

- Necrotising sialometaplasia is a benign, ulcerative lesion, usually located towards the back of the hard palate
- Probably caused by ischaemic necrosis of minor salivary glands in response to trauma

2.5 Question

How would you manage the patient?

Answer

- Incisional biopsy
- Analgesia
- Review in 2 weeks with histology

2.6 Question

Biopsy demonstrates lymphoma. How would you manage this?

Answer

- Referral to oncology/haematology
- Discussion at haematology MDT
- Head and neck CT: for evidence of lymphoma elsewhere and extent of lesion (Box D)
- Possibly full-body staging scans

2.7 Question

How would you treat the patient?

Answer

- Surgical excision followed by radiotherapy
- Treat systemically and await response
- If head and neck lesions cause local symptoms (i.e. compression related) then treat accordingly

Box A: Differential diagnosis of an oral cavity ulcer

- Malignant: squamous cell carcinoma, salivary gland cancer
- Idiopathic: recurrent aphthous ulceration
- Trauma
- Chemical: aspirin
- Infective: bacterial, viral
- Immunological: lichen planus, pemphigoid, Behçets. (vesiculobullous)
- Systemic: gastrointestinal, rheumatological
- Iatrogenic: nicorandil

Box B: Comprehensive examination of an oral lesion

End of the bed:
- Crusting of lips
- Rash

Inspection:
- Upper and lower lips
- Left and right buccal mucosa
- Dorsum of tongue with it protruded
- Ventral tongue with it elevated
- Hard palate
- Oropharyngeal tissues including soft palate

Palpation:
- Bimanual palpation of floor of mouth
- Lymph nodes

Transillumination:
- Fluid-filled lesions

Auscultation:
- Vascular lesions

Fibre optic visualisation:
- Visualise the oropharynx

Box C: Broad presentations of aphthous ulcers

- Minor: <5 mm wide, 1–5 at a time, last 1–2 weeks and heal without scarring
- Major: >10 mm wide, usually single, last 2–6 weeks and may heal with scarring
- Herpetiform: up to 50 ulcers of 1 mm size that can coalesce

Box D: Head and neck lymphoma

- Lymphoma may be nodal or extranodal
- The most frequent location of extranodal lymphoma in the head and neck is the palate
- Lymphoma usually appears as a nontender diffuse mass, which may ulcerate
- Many salivary gland lymphocytic infiltrates of the palate are usually non-Hodgkin B-cell lymphomas of mucosa-associated lymphoid tissue (MALT)

Further reading

Makepeace AR, Fermont DC, Bennett MH. Non-Hodgkin's lymphoma of the nasopharynx, paranasal sinus and palate. Clin Radiol 1989; 40:144–146.

Rice DH. Non inflammatory, non-neoplastic disorders of the salivary glands. Otolaryngol Clin North Am 1999; 32:835–843.

Short case 3: Fibrous dysplasia

The 20-year-old patient shown in the figure has presented with slowly growing fullness of the cheek lesion over last year.

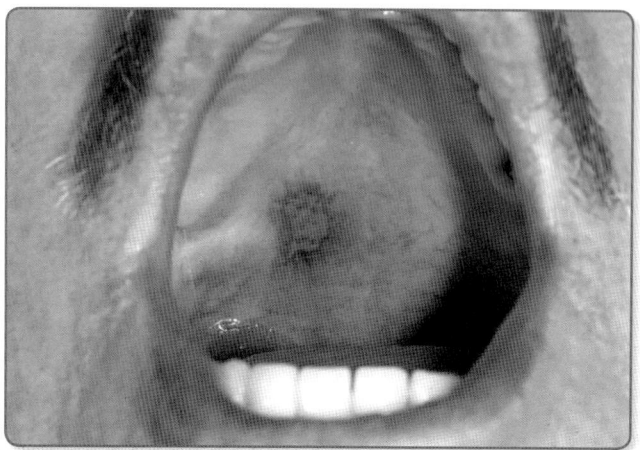

3.1 Question

What are the key points in the history?

Answer

- Swelling: duration, progression, unilateral or bilateral, pain
- Sensation: numbness
- Ocular symptoms: diplopia and vision
- Dental problems
- Nasal: obstruction and discharge
- General health: including drug history and allergies

3.2 Question

What are key points in the examination?

Answer

Extraoral:
- End of the bed: general health/sepsis, symmetry, syndromal
- Cheek: hard or soft tissue, objective measures of altered sensation
- Eyes: globe position, restricted movement
- Cervical lymph nodes

Intraoral:
- Cheek: intraoral swelling, obliteration of sulcus
- Parotid duct
- Teeth and gingivae

3.3 Question
Examination demonstrates firm swelling of the cheek with some altered sensation. How would you assess the patient further?

Answer
- OPG: identify a possible dental cause and potentially bone pathology
- Periapicals: to delineate dental pathology if unclear on an OPG
- CT: to relate potential bone pathology to adjacent structures
- Bone profile
- Nasal examination: intranasal (thudacums and endoscopy), Cottles test

3.4 Question
Please comment on the CT images?

Answer
- Axial and coronal slices demonstrate an abnormality in the left maxilla
- Poorly demarcated area of mixed radiolucency affecting bone around maxillary sinus
- Bone expansion but orbit and globe position appear unaffected
- Affects infraorbital area probably responsible for altered sensation

3.5 Question
What is the likely diagnosis?

Answer
- Ground glass appearance: hyperparathyroidism or fibrous osseous lesion (Box A)
- Most likely represents fibrous dysplasia (Box B)

3.6 Question
How would you manage the patient from here?

Answer
- Bone biopsy: intraoral vestibular approach
- Assessment of other bones: referral to orthopaedics if lesions outside of the head and neck suspected (Box C)
- Rule out associated syndromes: serum for PTH and ACTH (Box D)
- Cranial nerve examination

3.7 Question
Bone biopsy shows thin, irregular (Chinese character-like) bony trabeculae with a fibrotic marrow space. What does this mean and would you recommend any treatment?

Answer
- Biopsy result in keeping with fibrous dysplasia (Box E)

- Try not to treat in hope that it burns out
- If cheek swelling becomes prominent can be burred down
- Decompression of infraorbital nerve may be successful
- Medical treatment: bisphosphonates used for bone pain but no effect on progression

3.8 Question

The patient presents acutely to your clinic with rapid growth of her cheek. What are your concerns?

Answer
- Most likely represents an acute bleed
- Repeat CT imaging required
- A bleed into maxillary sinus should be self-limiting and can be managed conservatively

---

Box A: Types of fibro-cemento-osseous lesions

- Focal: periapical cemento-osseous dysplasia
- Generalised: florid cemento-osseous dysplasia
- Cementoblastoma
- Cemento ossifying fibroma
- Fibrous dysplasia

Box B: Pathology of fibrous dysplasia

- Rare non-neoplastic benign bone disease
- Abnormal proliferation of bone-forming mesenchyme
- Bone maturation stalls at the woven bone stage

Box C: Classification of fibrous dysplasia

- Monostotic: single bone (e.g. craniofacial only)
- Polyostotic: multiple bones (craniofacial + other)

Box D: McCune–Albright syndrome

Associated with Polyostotic fibrous dysplasia:
- Typically in girls with precocious puberty
- Café-au-lait macules
- Tumours of the pituitary gland
- Endocrine abnormalities: hyperthyroidism, cushings
- Cranial nerve palsies

> **Box E: Common presentations of craniofacial fibrous dysplasia**
> - Usually presents as an enlarging mass in the maxilla or mandible
> - Mass effect can cause cranial nerve compression, proptosis and malocclusion
> - Malignant transformation 0.5%
> - Usually progressive until about 30 years

Further reading

DiMeglio LA. Bisphosphonate therapy for fibrous dysplasia. Pediatr Endocrinol Rev 2007; 4: 440–445.

Macdonald-Jankowski DS, Li TK. Fibrous dysplasia in a Hong Kong community: the clinical and radiological features and outcomes of treatment. Dentomaxillofac Radiol 2009; 38:63–72.

Short case 4: Mucous membrane pemphigoid

The patient shown in the figure attends clinic complaining of sore gums, mouth ulcers and crusting of the lips.

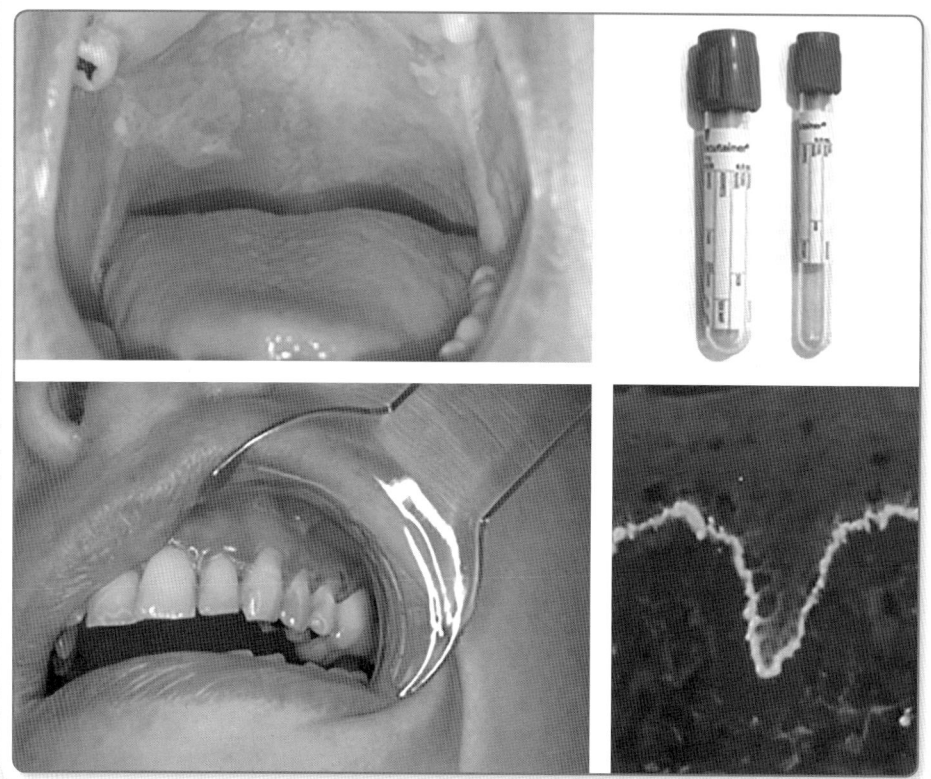

4.1 Question

What are the key points in the history?

Answer

- Duration of symptoms
- Eyes: discomfort, altered vision, grittiness
- Genital ulceration
- Skin lesions, usually head neck
- Other GIT symptoms suggestive of stenosis, dysphagia, hoarseness
- Previous treatment
- General medical health including allergies
- Drug history: recent changes in medication
- Social history: smoking

Short case 4 Mucous membrane pemphigoid

4.2 Question
How would you examine the patient?

Answer
Extraoral:
- Facial skin
- Skin elsewhere if lesions present
- Eyes

Intraoral:
- Lips, palate, buccal
- Gingivae: desquamative gingivitis
- Ulcers
- Scars

4.3 Question
Raw lesions and blisters are seen on both cheeks and tongue but the skin is normal. What is your differential diagnosis?

Answer
- Lichen planus
- Vesiculobullous disorder: pemphigus, pemphigoid, linear IgA bullous dermatosis
- Stephens–Johnson syndrome
- Herpetic gingivostomatitis
- Herpetiform recurrent aphthous ulceration
- Erythema multiforme minor

4.4 Question
The patient has only ever had symptoms in their mouth. How would you manage the patient from here?

Answer
- Biopsy of perilesional area that is not blistered, preserved for transport in formalin

4.5 Question
Biopsy demonstrates blistering and an inflammatory infiltrate along the basement membrane. What does the biopsy result signify and how would you manage this?

Answer
- The biopsy result is suspicious for a vesiculobullous disorder (Box A)
- Repeat biopsy: fresh sample for direct immunofluorescence (Box B)
- Blood test (red top bottle): indirect immunofluorescence

4.6 Question

Direct immunofluorescence shows separation at the basement membrane. What does the biopsy result signify and what treatment would you recommend based on the result?

Answer

- This likely represents mucous membrane pemphigoid (Box C)
- Referral to dermatology to asses for skin lesions
- Ophthalmology assessment: even if asymptomatic
- Start on topical steroids

4.7 Question

What drug and dose would you advise?

Answer

- Topical clobetasol propionate demonstrated to be more effective than systemic steroids in an RCT
- Tacrolimus ointment an alternative
- Reduce dose of oral steroids for flare ups (Box D)
- Liaise with dermatology about steroid sparing drugs (e.g. azathioprine, mycofenalate) although their effectiveness has been questioned

---

Box A: Pemphigus and pemphigoid

- Group of autoimmune blistering diseases affecting the skin and less commonly the mucous membranes and eyes
- IgG antibodies and C3 complement target hemidesmosomes along basement membrane (pemphigoid) or between epithelial cells (pemphigus)
- Pemphigoid bullae tend to last longer because cleavage is deeper as in basement membrane
- Pemphigus is more severe and is potentially fatal so needs to be treated more aggressively
- Both can produce desquamative gingivitis
- Nikolsky's sign: not used in practice to differentiate between pemphigus vulgaris (present) and bullous pemphigoid (absent)

Box B: Concept behind immunofluorescence

- Fluorescent molecule attached to an antibody
- Antibody recognises the target molecule (antigen)
- The attached fluorophore can be detected via fluorescent light microscopy

> **Box C: Interpreting biopsy results**
> - Standard biopsy: blistering and inflammatory infiltrate along basement membrane (pemphigoid) or between epithelial cells (pemphigus)
> - Direct immunofluorescence: IgG antibody and/or C3 complement along basement membrane (pemphigoid) or between epithelial cells (pemphigus)
> - Indirect immunofluorescence: circulating serum IgG autoantibodies

> **Box D: Treatment of pemphigus and pemphigoid**
> - If unsure which disorder it is initially treat aggressively with high dose systemic steroids as pemphigus can be fatal
> - Pemphigus: systemic immunosuppression with steroids and steroid sparing agents (azathioprine, myclophenolate, cyclophosphamide)
> - Pemphigoid: generally can treat with topical steroids, tacrolimus ointment. More severe disease will need systemic treatment as per pemphigus
> - Tetracycline and nicotinamde (vitamin B3)

Further reading

Joly P, Roujeau JC, Benichou J, et al. A comparison of oral and topical corticosteroids in patients with bullous pemphigoid. N Engl J Med 2002; 346:321–327.

Kirtschig G, Middleton P, Bennett C, et al. Interventions for bullous pemphigoid. Cochrane Database Syst Rev 2010:CD002292.

Short case 5: Oral lichen planus

The patient shown in the figure has been referred by their dentist who is concerned about an ulcerated white area in their cheek.

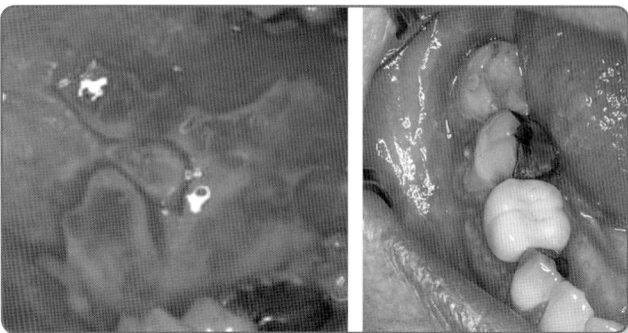

5.1 Question
What are the key points in the history?

Answer
- Lesion: progression, pain
- Previous lesions: oral, skin
- Previous treatment: including biopsies
- Associated structures: swelling, numbness, weakness, limitation in mouth opening
- General medical health
- Drug history
- Social history: smoking, alcohol, stress, family support

5.2 Question
What are the key points in the examination?

Answer

Extraoral:
- General health
- Cheek: swelling, skin changes
- Lymphadenopathy

Intraoral:
- Single or multiple areas
- Lesion type: ulceration, erosion, bullae, striation
- Induration or fixation to underlying structures including mouth opening

5.3 Question
You note a buccal white patch with ulceration including the attached gingivae. What is the likely diagnosis?

Answer
- Probably represents erosive lichen planus with associated desquamative gingivitis (Box A)
- Differential diagnoses of oral epithelial lesions include malignant, potentially premalignant and benign (Box B)

5.4 Question
How would you manage the patient further?

Answer
- Incisional biopsy to confirm diagnosis
- Address potentially contributing factors (Box C)

5.5 Question
How would you perform the biopsy?

Answer
- Type: scalpel
- Width: include most representative area
- Depth: full mucosal thickness
- Consent: parotid duct damage, numbness, scar, pain

5.6 Question
The biopsy confirms lichen planus (Box B). Mild dysplasia is noted. How would you manage this further?

Answer
- Repeat biopsy to confirm dysplasia and monitor
- Pain relievers: benzydamine mouthwash, oral analgesia
- Topical steroids: used for 2 weeks when symptomatic: betamethasone, prednisolone, clobetasol, fluticasone
- Oral steroids: given as a reducing dose if severe
- Address risk factors for dysplasia (e.g. smoking) and potentially contributing factors to LP (Box C)

5.7 Question
Repeat biopsy comes back with no dysplasia. The patient wants to know what the chances of the area becoming malignant are?

Answer
- Several molecular alterations implicating pre-neoplastic changes are detectable in OLP
- No firm biological pathway from OLP to malignancy has been established
- Erosive, atrophic and plaque subtypes have the highest transformation rates
- This patient with erosive LP probably has a realistic lifetime risk of 1–3%

5.8 Question

How would you follow the patient up?

Answer
- No guidelines currently exist
- Patients are generally followed up every 6 months
- Asymptomatic patients and lower risk clinical manifestations (e.g. reticular) can be discharged after 2 years
- Many clinicians recommend follow-up of all other presentations for life – this can be with the patient's own dentist

---

Box A: Clinical subtypes of lichen planus

- Reticular (80%): raised white striations
- Erosive (10%): painful, slow healing ulcers/erosions, desquamative gingivitis
- Atrophic: red atrophic areas, desquamative gingivitis
- Plaque: raised white patches (leukoplakia)
- Papular: small clumps of white papules
- Bullous: fluid-filled vesicles

Box B: Differential diagnosis of buccal white patch with ulceration

- Malignant: squamous cell carcinoma
- Potentially malignant: leukoplakia, hyperplastic candidiasis, submucous fibrosis
- Immunological: lichen planus/reaction, pemphigoid, pemphigus
- Infective: candidiasis
- Inflammatory: smokers keratosis
- Traumatic: frictional keratosis

Box C: Factors potentially contributing to lichen planus

- Dental materials: amalgam, gold
- Stress
- Autoimmunity including diabetes
- Food allergies
- Drugs: NSAIDs
- Preservatives in toothpaste: sodium lauryl sulphate
- Infectious agents: hepatitis C association described

Further reading

Awadallah M, Idle M, Patel K, Kademani D. Management update of potentially premalignant oral epithelial lesions. Oral Surg Oral Med Oral Pathol Oral Radiol 2018; 125:628–636.

Greaney L, Brennan PA, Kerawala C, et al. Why should I follow up my patients with oral lichen planus and lichenoid reactions? Br J Oral Maxillofac Surg 2014; 52:291–293.

Thomson PJ, McCaul J, Ridout F, Hutchison I. To treat...or not to treat? Clinicians' views on the management of oral potentially malignant disorders. Br J Oral Maxillofac Surg 2015; 53: 1027–1031.

Short case 6: Oral pigmentation and mucosal melanoma

The patient shown in this figure attended their dentist worried about a black spot in their mouth.

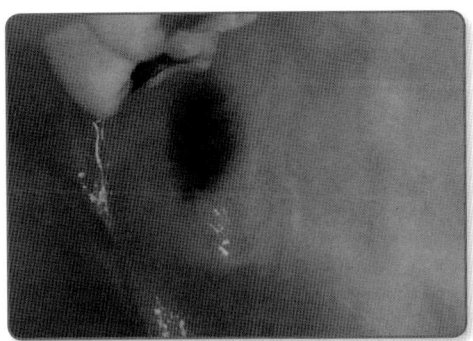

6.1 Question

What are the key points in the history?

Answer

- Onset of pigmentation, duration, progression (e.g. starting to ulcerate)
- Localised or diffuse (Box A)
- Pigmentation elsewhere in mouth or body
- Previous dental treatment or extractions in area
- Medical history and allergies
- Drug history (Box B)
- Lymphadenopathy
- Immunosuppression

6.2 Question

What are the key points in the examination?

Answer

- Localised or diffuse (Box A)
- Perioral pigmentation: Peutz–Jeghers
- Adjacent restored or extracted tooth: amalgam tattoo
- Blanching of lesion under pressure: vascular malformation

6.3 Question

You only find one affected area. What is the differential diagnosis of a single lesion?

Answer

- Most likely amalgam tattoo: adjacent large amalgam, extracted teeth (Box A)
- Unable to definitively rule out melanoma

6.4 Question

How would you manage the patient?

Answer

- Excisional biopsy: with care not to damage adjacent parotid duct orifice
- Incisional biopsy: may assist in suspicious small lesions (<0.5 cm) as can be difficult to locate for later further resection

6.5 Question

Histology reports a melanocytic naevus but the patient is worried as they are sure it was not present a few years ago. How would you manage the patient?

Answer

- Reassurance that this represents a benign local proliferation of melanocytes
- Explain that they are not always present at birth
- Discharge with no follow-up

6.6 Question

If the histology had demonstrated atypical melanocytes invading the lamina propria, what does this signify and how would you manage this?

Answer

- Represents oral mucosal melanoma (Box C)
- Review histology for excision margins
- Stage with MRI head, neck and chest: localised, regional, distant spread
- Discuss at skin MDT

6.7 Question

The lesion was excised with clear margins (>1 cm) and no local or distant spread was found. How would you manage this?

Answer

- Evidence supporting management of oral mucosal melanoma is lacking
- Lesions spread radially so wider excision is generally recommended but this remains contentious even if margins are clear
- N0 neck: no evidence to support neck dissection (Box D)
- N+ neck: surgery for regional control and symptom relief

6.8 Question

Would you give any adjuvant treatment?

Answer

- NICE 2016 recommends radiotherapy even in absence of metastasis
- For small lesions excised with good margins, radiotherapy not recommended
- Chemotherapy is used for distant metastasis but there is little evidence to support this

Short case 6 Oral pigmentation and mucosal melanoma

Box A: Causes of oral mucosal pigmentation

Localised:
- Idiopathic
- Melanotic naevus
- Kaposi's sarcoma
- Amalgam tattoo
- Vascular malformations
- Mucosal melanoma

Diffuse:
- Racial
- Addisons
- Peutz–Jeghers
- Heavy metal poisoning
- Smokers melanosis
- Drug induced

Box B: Drugs most commonly causing mucosal pigmentation

- Antimalarials: quinacrine, chloroquine, hydroxychloroquine
- Zidovudine
- Tetracyclines
- Chlorpromazine
- Oral contraceptives

Box C: Oral mucosal melanoma

- Rare: 1% of all melanomas
- Far more aggressive than skin melanoma
- More inclined to metastasise into regional and distant sites or recur
- Five-year survival rate 10–15%
- Exposure to sunlight not an aetiological factor
- Peak incidence is 60–80 years old
- 20% local metastases at presentation, 10% distant metastases
- Radiotherapy and chemotherapy are used despite strong evidence to support it

Box D: Management of the neck in oral mucosal melanoma

- N1: Therapeutic neck dissection
- N0: Neck dissection not recommended
- SNLB: insufficient information to make recommendation on

Further reading

Cancer of the upper aerodigestive tract: assessment and management in people aged 16 and over. NICE guideline [NG36] Published date: February 2016 Last updated: June 2018.

Short case 7: Oral white patch and premalignancy

The patient shown in this figure is concerned about a white patch on their tongue.

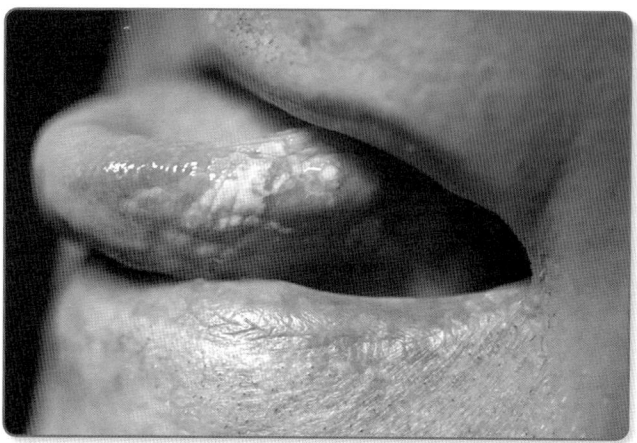

7.1 Question

What are the pertinent points in the history?

Answer

- Lesion: duration, progression, trauma
- Previous lesions or biopsies
- Associated symptoms: swallowing, sensation, otalgia, dysphonia, odynophagia, dysphagia
- Past medical history including previous head neck cancer
- Drug history: immunosuppression
- Social: smoking, alcohol, betel quid
- Family history
- Performance status

7.2 Question

What are the key points in the examination?

Answer

- Site: high risk lateral tongue FOM, association with structures (e.g. nerves, duct orifice)
- Size: incisional versus excisional biopsy
- Appearance: colour (leukoplakia, erythroplakia, mixed), homogeneous, erosive, speckled
- Feel: induration, attachment to underlying structures
- Associated structures: sensation and movement of tongue
- Cervical lymphadenopathy

7.3 Question

The area does not rub off. What is the differential diagnosis of homogeneous leukoplakia?

Answer

- Traumatic keratosis
- Lichen planus
- Chronic hyper plastic candidiasis (Box A)

7.4 Question

On examination the lesion shown in the figure is 3 cm in diameter. How would you manage the lesion?

Answer

- Incisional biopsy: down to muscle
- Address risk factors (Box B)

7.5 Question

Incisional biopsy demonstrates moderate dysplasia (Box C). How will you manage this?

Answer

- A recent review of surgeons practice on moderate dysplasia showed 1/3 watch and wait, 1/3 perform cold steel excision and 1/3 perform laser excision
- A lesion of this size and location can be excised with relatively small morbidity with a 5-mm margin

7.6 Question

Excisional biopsy demonstrates moderate dysplasia but has field change to the edge of the biopsy specimen. How will you manage this and what are the risks of each?

Answer

- Further excision and/or Lugol's iodine or frozen sections: risk of further incomplete excision, greater morbidity
- Surveillance: risk of malignant transformation
- Laser vaporisation: no margins available in biopsy specimen to ensure complete excision

7.7 Question

The patient asks what the risk of malignant transformation is if you did not perform further excision. How would you respond?

Answer

- A homogeneous white lesion with moderate dysplasia on the lateral border of the tongue has a range of 20–50% risk over 5 years should be advised
- Huge variations in published rates are reported (Box C)

7.8 Question

How would you follow-up the patient if you did not perform further excision?

Answer

- No guidelines currently exist
- Follow-up every 4 months would be prudent
- Clinical photographs should be provided to patient and dentist
- Smoking cessation can reduce lesions by 60%

Box A: Differential diagnosis of a tongue white patch

- Traumatic: frictional keratosis
- Infective: candidiasis, hairy leukoplakia
- Malignant: SCC
- Potentially malignant: leukoplakia
- Inflammatory: smokers keratosis, lichen planus

Box B: Poor prognostic factors for malignant transformation of leukoplakia

- Location: floor of mouth, ventral tongue
- Appearance: exophytic, erythematous, speckled
- Single lesion: multiple lesions better prognosis
- Degree of dysplasia: moderate or severe
- Social: smoking, alcohol, betel nut
- Male > female
- Smoking status and transformation is controversial
- Nonsmokers with dysplasia may have worse outcomes

Box C: Some 5-year transformation rates of white patches

- Site: lateral tongue (53%), buccal (29%), floor of mouth (8%)
- Dysplasia: mild (16%), moderate (24%), severe (33%)
- Appearance: homogeneous (15%), nonhomogeneous (40%)

Further reading

Ho MW, Risk JM, Woolgar JA, et al. The clinical determinants of malignant transformation in oral epithelial dysplasia. Oral Oncol 2012; 48:969–976.

Kuribayashi Y, Tsushima F, Morita KI, et al. Long-term outcome of non-surgical treatment in patients with oral leukoplakia. Oral Oncol 2015; 51:1020–1025.

Mehanna HM, Rattay T, Smith J, McConkey CC. Treatment and follow-up of oral dysplasia – a systematic review and meta-analysis. Head Neck 2009; 31:1600–1609.

Thomson PJ, McCaul J, Ridout F, Hutchison I. To treat or not to treat? Clinicians' views on the management of oral potentially malignant disorders. Br J Oral Maxillofac Surg 2015; 53: 1027–1031.

Short case 8: Osteoradionecrosis in the mandible

The patient shown in the figure complains of a sore mouth and exposed bone after a tooth extraction.

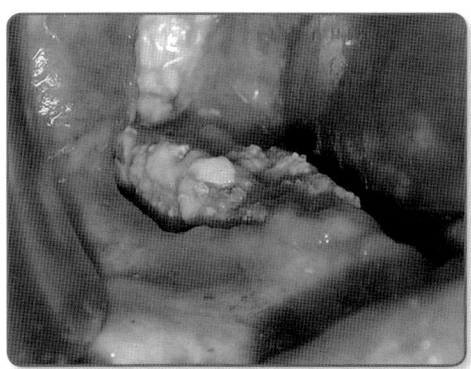

8.1 Question
Describe the key points in the history?

Answer
- Duration since extraction
- Pain
- Progression
- Other complications post extraction
- Reason for extraction: caries, previous infections
- Risk factors (Box A)
- General health: immunosuppression
- Drug history: those causing MRONJ
- Social history: smoking

8.2 Question
This patient had Intensity-modulated radiotherapy (IMRT) for tonsillar carcinoma. What are the key points in the examination?

Answer

Extraoral:
- General health
- Swelling and erythema
- Cutaneous sinus (fistula)

Intraoral:
- Exposed bone: extent, sequestration
- Overlying mucosa: mucosal dehiscence, erythema, fetor
- Occlusion: pathological fracture

8.3 Question

What is the likely diagnosis?

Answer

This patient probably has ORN (Box B). The most commonly used definition of ORN is: exposed, irradiated, nonhealing bone of at least 3 months duration without evidence of tumor recurrence

8.4 Question

What baseline investigations would you request?

Answer

- OPG and peripaicals: dental and periodontal pathology, prognosis of existing teeth
- CT: extent of necrosis, pathological fracture, lymphadenopathy
- Incisional biopsy: to ensure not malignant

8.5 Question

How would you manage this patient who has a 2-cm painless defect?

Answer

- Management depends on combating theories of ORN development (Box C)
- Notani staging: used in mandibular disease to guide treatment (Boxes D and E) but this staging is of little use in maxilla and does not include pain
- Prevention: leave out denture, oral hygiene, avoid extractions (root canal treatment), low dose oral doxycycline if repeated infections, steroids have been suggested
- Treatment: oral antibiotics (usually amoxicillin or bone penetrance antibiotic such as clindamycin) for exacerbations, sequestrotomy

8.6 Question

Is there anything else you can give to treat established ORN?

Answer

- Hyperbaric oxygen (HBO): current evidence for efficacy is debated and results of ongoing HOPON (prevention) and DAHANCE (treatment) trials are awaited
- PENTOCLO: pentoxifylline, tocopherol and clodronate: efficacy is debated. NICE guidelines recommend for trial purposes only
- Bone resection, saucerisation, sequestrectomy

8.7 Question

The patient asks if she should have had HBO prior to the extraction?

Answer
- Limited evidence exists to support giving HBO around the time of tooth extraction in at-risk patients
- Not current practice in the UK

8.8 Question
The patient asks if she should have had her at-risk teeth extracted prior to starting radiotherapy.

Answer
- Preradiotherapy extractions do not appear to reduce the risk of developing ORN

Box A: Risk factors for developing ORN

- Radiotherapy dose >60 Gy
- IMRT better (5% chance developing instead of 7% with conventional)
- Additional chemotherapy
- Trauma: extractions, denture irritation, biopsy
- Poor oral hygiene
- Immunodeficiency
- Malnutrition
- Smoking

Box B: Differential diagnosis of exposed bone

- Osteonecrosis: MRONJ, ORN
- Osteomyelitis
- Infection: osteomyelitis
- Neoplastic: recurrent SCC, metastasis

Box C: Proposed theories behind osteoradionecrosis

- Meyer: chronic infection – basis of antibiotics
- Marx: hypovascularity, hypocellularity and hypoxia – basis of hyperbaric oxygen
- Delanian: endothelial cell damage-free radical activation of inflammatory cytokine basis of PENTOCLO

Box D: Notani classification of mandibular ORN based upon an OPG radiograph

- Grade 1: confined to alveolar bone
- Grade 2: above level of IA nerve
- Grade 3: below the IA canal, +/− fistula or pathological fracture

> **Box E: Treatment of mandibular ORN based upon the Notani classification**
> - Grade 1: chlorhexidine mouthwash, antibiotics when required, consider PENTOCLO
> - Grade 2: consider sequestrotomy and mucosal closure, consider HBO
> - Grade 3: consider segmental resection

Further reading

Bennett MH, Feldmeier J, Hampson N, et al. Hyperbaric oxygen therapy for the treatment of the late effects of radiotherapy. Cochrane Database Syst Rev 2016; 4:CD005005.

Costa DA, Costa TP, Netto EC, et al. New perspectives on the conservative management of osteoradionecrosis of the mandible: A literature review. Head Neck 2016; 38:1708–1716.

Dhanda J, Pasquier D, Newman L, et al. Current Concepts in Osteoradionecrosis after Head and Neck Radiotherapy. Clin Oncol (R Coll Radiol) 2016; 28:459–466.

Short case 9: Gingival mass

This patient is complaining of a lump growing on their upper gingivae.

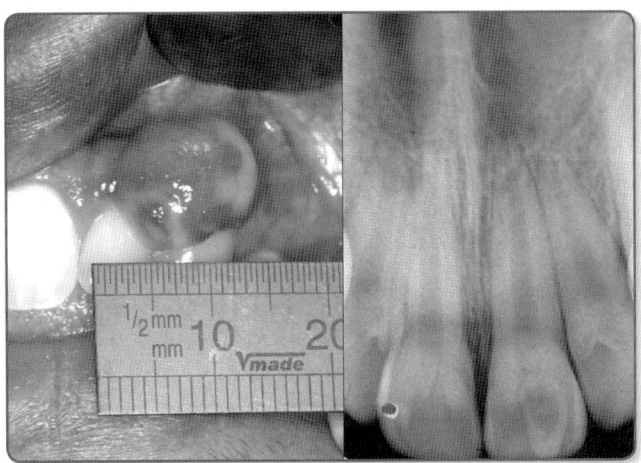

9.1 Question
What are the key points in the history?

Answer

- Isolated lump/swelling or generalised
- Lump: progression, regression, previous occurrences
- Lumps elsewhere in body: neck, axilla
- Associated symptoms: pain, bleeding
- General health, pregnancy
- Drug history (Box A)
- Social history: smoking, alcohol

9.2 Question
The patient takes phenytoin for epilepsy but is otherwise well. What are the key points in the examination?

Answer

Extraoral:
- General health
- Lip: swelling, erythema

Intraoral:
- Discrete lesion/regional/generalised (Box B)
- Lesion: colour, shape, consistency (hard/fluctuant), attached gingiva, submucosal
- Dental health of associated teeth, vitality, tenderness to percussion, caries
- Periodontal health

9.3 Question

Examination demonstrates a discrete pedunculated lesion on the gingivae. What is the likely diagnosis?

Answer

- Most likely a pyogenic granuloma
- Differentials should include a fibrous epulis, vascular malformation, periodontal abscess or giant cell granuloma (Box B)

9.4 Question

How would you manage the patient further?

Answer

- Periapical radiograph: periapical and periodontal pathology
- OPG: rule out underlying bone lesion, bone profile (PTH, Ca, Po)
- Vitality testing of adjacent teeth
- Excision of lesion under local anaesthesia, excisional or incisional biopsy

9.5 Question

How will you perform the biopsy?

Answer

- Local anaesthesia.
- Scalpel excision with 1–2 mm margin
- Diathermy
- Simple postoperative oral analgesia
- Benzydamine mouthwash

9.6 Question

How would you advise the patient ahead of the biopsy?

Answer

- Complications: bleeding, gingival recession
- Further treatment may be necessary depending on histology result
- Probability of malignancy rare (1%)

9.7 Question

The lesion is diagnosed as a pyogenic granuloma (Box C). How will you explain this diagnosis to the patient?

Answer

- Overgrowth of gingiva in response to local irritants
- Multiple causes, including pregnancy (Box B)
- Noncancerous or related to pus (a misnomer), but may recur

9.8 Question

How will you follow-up the patient?

Answer

- Patient should be reviewed in 3–4 months for gingival healing
- Patient should visit their dentist in the interim
- Need to maintain strict periodontal health

Box A: Drug-induced gingival enlargement

- Anticonvulsants: phenytoin, lamotrigine
- Immunosuppressants: ciclosporin, tacrolimus
- Calcium channel blockers: nifedipine, felodipine, amlodipine, verapamil

---

Box B: Differential diagnosis of gingival lumps

- Discrete lesion: Pyogenic granuloma, fibrous epulis, periodontal abscess, vascular malformation, focal fibrous dysplasia, peripheral giant cell granuloma
- Regional (multiple teeth): mouth breathing, leukaemia/lymphoma
- Generalised: drug-induced (Box B), Wegeners granulomatosis, Crohn's, sarcoidosis

---

Box C: Causes of pyogenic granuloma

- Low grade local irritation: periodontal or periapical disease
- Traumatic
- Hormones: progesterone, oestrogen
- Drugs

Further reading

Babu B, Hallikeri K. Reactive lesions of oral cavity: A retrospective study of 659 cases. J Indian Soc Periodontol 2017; 21:258–263.

Saravana GH. Oral pyogenic granuloma: a review of 137 cases. Br J Oral Maxillofac Surg 2009; 47:318–319.

Tamiolakis P, Chatzopoulou E, Frakouli F, et al. Localized gingival enlargements. A clinicopathological study of 1187 cases. Med Oral Patol Oral Cir Bucal 2018; 23:e320–e325.

Short case 10: Keratocystic odontogenic tumour

The patient with the radiograph shown in the figure presents to you in clinic.

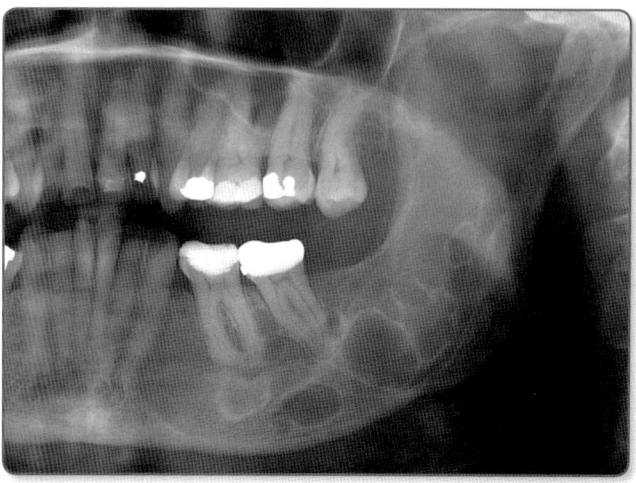

10.1 Question
What is the differential diagnosis?

Answer

Simplified differential diagnosis of a multilocular radiolucency at the angle of mandible includes:
- Tumour: ameloblastoma, KOT, odontogenic myxoma
- Cyst: dentigerous cyst
- Other: giant cell lesion, vascular malformation

10.2 Question
How would you clinically assess the patient?

Answer
- History
- Examination
- Investigations

10.3 Question
What are the key features in the history?

Answer
- Rapidity of growth
- Skin sensation (nerve involvement)
- Occlusion (pathological fracture)

- Family history of Gorlin's syndrome (Box A)
- Previous treatment

10.4 Question

What are the key examination features?

Answer

- Tooth mobility
- Pathological fracture
- Expansion

10.5 Question

How would you investigate such new lesions?

Answer

- OPG: lesions are most commonly found in the posterior mandible (Box B)
- CT: delineate soft tissue invasion, calcification of falx cerebri
- Chest X-ray: bifid or missing ribs, fused vertebrae
- Open biopsy: for histology

10.6 Question

How would you undertake the biopsy?

Answer

Depends on whether lesion is cystic or solid:
- Cystic: take sample of lining and place a grommet to decompress
- Solid: take a sample of lesion and close mucosa primarily (it may represent an ameloblastoma)

10.7 Question

What histopathological features would you expect?

Answer

- Benign but locally aggressive neoplasm (WHO 2005 classification)
- Lining is keratinised stratified squamous epithelium
- 'Daughter cysts' bud off from walls
- Two main histological variants reflect clinical activity and management (Box D)

10.8 Question

How would you treat the lesion?

Answer

- Main options are either enucleation alone, or marsupialisation followed by enucleation
- Marsupialisation prior to enucleation allows for bony infill to reduce risk of pathological fractureEnucleation is performed by curettage (assisted by a

drill) followed by treatment of walls of lesion with Carnoy's (Box E), liquid nitrogen, or 5-fluorouracil
- Electrocautery used to excise mucosal breaches

10.9 Question
How would you follow the patient up?

Answer
- Recurrences can occur late
- Follow-up yearly for 10 years

10.10 Question
What is the risk of recurrence following different types of treatment?

Answer
- Curettage: 19%
- Enucleation alone: 29%
- Enucleation and Carnoy's: 2%
- 'Radical' enucleation: 17%
- Enucleation and cryotherapy: 31%
- Marsupialisation: 24% (Box D)
- Resection: 0%

Box A: Key features of Gorlin's syndrome

Major criteria:
- Multiple basal cell carcinomas (BCCs)
- Multiple KOT
- Palmar or plantar pits
- Calcification of falx cerebri
- Family history

Minor criteria:
- Bifid ribs
- Vertebral anomalies
- Increased head circumference
- Frontal bossing
- Hypertelorism

Box B: Key radiological features of KOT

- Generally posterior mandible
- Multilocular radiolucency
- Aggressive appearance
- Erosion of mandible and teeth
- Displacement of third molar tooth

Box C: Marsupialisation of KOT

- Highly controversial if used alone and most effective in reducing size of lesion for further surgery
- A case series (Pogrel et al. in 2004) concluded that marsupialisation alone can produce complete resolution but the findings were partly retracted in 2005 following recurrence in some cases

Box D: Histological features of KOT

- Parakeratinised: ↑ aggression, ↑ daughter cysts, ↑ recurrence, Gorlin's syndrome
- Orthokeratinised: ↓ aggression

Box E: Carnoy's solution

- Comprised of absolute alcohol, chloroform and acetic acid
- Ribbon gauze or cotton wool pledgers are soaked in the solution and applied to the cavity for 3 minutes before rinsing
- Risks are damage to the lining of the maxillary sinus or exposed nerves
- Procuring this solution is challenging and therefore it is rarely used

Further reading

Blanas N, Freund B, Schwartz M, Furst IM. Systematic review of the treatment and prognosis of the odontogenic keratocyst. Oral Surg Oral Med Oral Pathol Oral Radiol Endod 2000; 90:553–558.

Pogrel MA, Jordan RC. Marsupialization as a definitive treatment for the odontogenic keratocyst. J Oral Maxillofac Surg 2004; 62:651–655.

Stoelinga P. Long-term follow-up on keratocysts treated according to a defined protocol. Int J Oral Maxillofac Surg 2001; 30:14–25.

Short case 11: Calcifying epithelial odontogenic tumour

One of your junior doctors is seeing the patient shown in this figure in your emergency follow-up clinic with a growing lump on their gum.

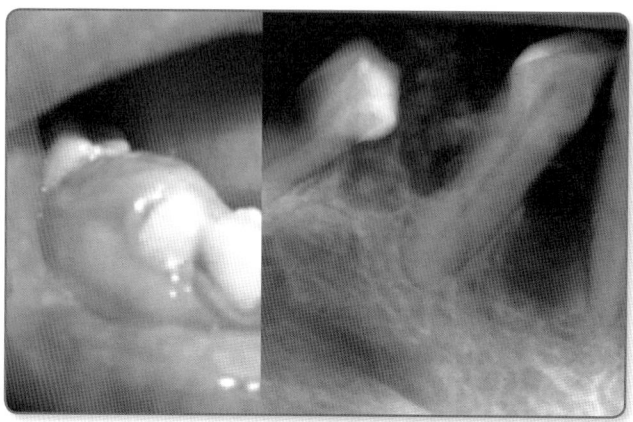

11.1 Question
What are the key points in the history?

Answer

- Lump: speed of growth, bleeding, pain, loosening teeth, lip numbness
- Associated symptoms: recent dental treatment or problems
- General health and fitness for surgery
- Drug history

11.2 Question
What are the pertinent points in the examination?

Answer

- Extraoral: general health, mandibular swelling, lip numbness, cervical lymphadenopathy
- Intraoral: swelling size, shape, colour, pulsatility, tooth mobility, periodontal disease

11.3 Question
How would you investigate this further?

Answer

- Periapical: dental and periodontal pathology
- OPG: associated bone changes, extent of any lesion
- Incisional biopsy

11.4 Question
Describe the appearance of this radiograph systematically (Box A)?

Answer
- Site: periapical radiograph of the mandibular right premolar region
- Size: lesion approximately 15–20 mm associated with the canine and second premolar teeth
- Shape: unilocular (more common in the maxilla)/multilocular, coronal clustering and invading soft tissues
- Outline: diffuse and poorly corticated
- Relative radiodensity: mixed radiolucency with internal radiopacities present
- Adjacent structures: no root resorption, lateral incisor displaced, caries in premolar

11.5 Question
What is the differential diagnosis?

Answer
- Poorly corticated area of mixed radiolucency (Box B)
- Not a discrete radiolucent lesion
- May represent odontogenic or nonodontogenic causes (Box C)

11.6 Question
The histology demonstrates a calcifying epithelial odontogenic tumour (Boxes D and E)

Answer
- Benign odontogenic tumour but locally aggressive
- Resection with 5 mm margins
- Wait for clear margins before considering reconstruction

11.7 Question
How would you reconstruct the area?

Answer
- Options dependent on patient's wishes and general health
- A nonvascularised bone graft (autograft, xenografts) followed by implants for prosthesis retention would be the recommended option

11.8 Question
How would you follow-up the patient and what is the incidence of recurrence?

Answer
- Follow-up every 6 months for 5 years
- OPG or CBCT yearly for 5 years
- Recurrence of 12–20% is quoted

> **Box A: Systematic description of a radiolucent lesion will aid diagnosis**
> - Site: anatomical location
> - Size: in millimetres
> - Shape: unilocular, multilocular, scalloped
> - Outline: well corticated, diffuse, punched out
> - Relative radiodensity: compared to surrounding structures, internal radiopacities
> - Effects on adjacent surrounding structures: root resorption, fracture, tooth displacement
> - Association with teeth, presence of impaction

> **Box B: Lesions of mixed radiolucency affecting the bone**
> - Odontogenic: calcifying epithelial odontogenic tumour (CEOT), adenomatoid odontogenic tumour
> - Nonodontogenic: fibro cemento-osseous lesions, Paget's disease, osteomyelitis

> **Box C: Lesions that can present as a cyst-like radiolucency**
> - Odontogenic cysts: radicular (or residual) cyst, lateral periodontal cyst, dentigerous cyst.
> - Nonodontogenic cysts: nasopalatine duct cyst
> - Odontogenic tumours: odontogenic keratocyst, ameloblastoma, calcifying epithelial odontogenic tumour
> - Nonodontogenic tumours: osteosarcoma, squamous cell carcinoma, multiple myeloma, lymphoma
> - Others: giant cell lesions, fibro-cemento-osseous lesions, Stafne's bone cavity

> **Box D: Calcifying epithelial odontogenic tumour**
> - 'Pindborg tumour', named after the first person to describe it
> - WHO classification 2005: a locally aggressive tumour and not a cyst
> - Types: central (within bone), peripheral (soft tissue swelling)
> - Clear cell variant (8% of cases) is more aggressive and more likely to recur

> **Box E: Radiological appearance of calcifying epithelial odontogenic tumours**
> - Uni or multilocular radiolucency
> - Small radiopacities within it ('driven-snow')
> - Root resorption or divergence

Further reading

Anavi Y, Kaplan I, Citir M, et al. Clear-cell variant of calcifying epithelial odontogenic tumor: clinical and radiographic characteristics. Oral Surg Oral Med Oral Pathol Oral Radiol Endod 2003; 95:332–339.

Chrcanovic BR, Gomez RS. Calcifying epithelial odontogenic tumor: An updated analysis of 339 cases reported in the literature. J Craniomaxillofac Surg 2017; 45:1117–1123.

Long case 12: Recurrent multicystic ameloblastoma

This 70-year-old patient is returning to clinic for her histology results. She recalls having a similar lesion operated on 20 years ago.

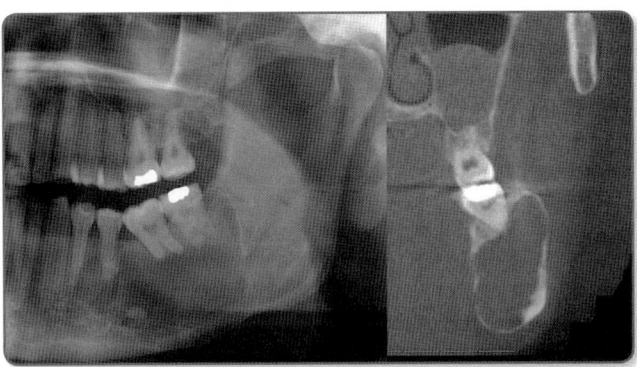

12.1 Question
How would you assess this patient's radiograph?

Answer
- Introduce yourself, clean your hands and obtain consent to assess
- Tailor your assessment to the potential diagnoses of a unilocular mandibular radiolucency (Box A)

12.2 Question
What are the key points in the history?

Answer
- Presenting complaint: swelling, altered sensation, tooth loosening
- Previous treatment: enucleation of lesion in same area 20 years ago
- Medical fitness for surgery

12.3 Question
How would you examine the patient?

Answer
- Extraoral: bony expansion, lip numbness, pathological fracture
- Intraoral: tooth mobility, tongue numbness

12.4 Question
How would you investigate the patient further?

Answer
- OPG
- CT
- Histology

12.5 Question

What can you see in the radiograph?

Answer

- Unilocular radiolucency in the mandibular body (Box B)
- Tooth resorption suggestive of an aggressive lesion

12.6 Question

CT demonstrates a multilocular lesion (Box C). Histology comes back as ameloblastoma (Box D). What is the overall diagnosis?

Answer

- Multicystic ameloblastoma
- Likely recurrence from previous incomplete surgery

12.7 Question

How would you treat this patient?

Answer

- Summarise findings: unsuspected
- Curative surgical treatment: 1 cm margin necessitating segmental resection
- Reconstruction: nonvascularised cortico-cancellous block graft, heavy profile prebent plate, osseointegrated implants
- Potential complications: infection, numbness, plate fracture, incomplete removal
- Treatment options for the nonsurgically fit patient: enucleation and a heavy profile plate only, accepting that though recurrence likely, will take many years
- Potential for malignant transformation

Box A: Concept of the oral medicine long case

- A 15-minute assessment likely encompassing the structure above
- An oral medicine long case is unusual
- It would most likely involve a more complex pathology, such as a vesiculobullous disorder or a bone lesion requiring surgery

---

Box B: Differential diagnosis of a unilocular radiolucency

- Odontogenic cysts: radicular, dentigerous, residual, calcifying odontogenic cyst
- Odontogenic tumours: unicystic ameloblastoma
- Nonodontogenic: Stafne's bone cyst, vascular malformation

> **Box C: Differential diagnosis of a multilocular radiolucency**
> - Odontogenic cysts: dentigerous cyst
> - Odontogenic tumours: ameloblastoma, keratocyst (OKCT), myxoma
> - Nonodontogenic lesions: giant cell lesion, vascular malformation

> **Box D: Radiological appearance of ameloblastoma guides clinical nature**
> - Unicystic: less aggressive and more common in children
> - Multicystic (solid): more aggressive, may damage teeth or cause paraesthesia
> - Peripheral

Further reading

Effiom OA, Ogundana OM1, Akinshipo AO, Akintoye SO. Ameloblastoma: current etiopathological concepts and management. Oral Dis 2018; 24:307–316.

Parmar S, Al-Qamachi L, Aga H. Ameloblastomas of the mandible and maxilla. Curr Opin Otolaryngol Head Neck Surg 2016; 24:148–154.

Chapter 8

Temporomandibular joint surgery

SHORT CASES

1. Temporomandibular joint (TMJ) history
2. Temperomandibular joint examination
3. Osteoarthritis (OA) of the TMJ
4. Synovial chondromatosis and MRI
5. Closed lock and MRI
6. SPECT interpretation
7. Alloplastic TMJ replacement
8. Recurrent TMJ dislocation

LONG CASE

9. TMJ ankylosis

Short case 1: Temporomandibular joint (TMJ) history

This is the first consultation for a patient referred by their dentist with suspected temperomandibular joint dysfunction.

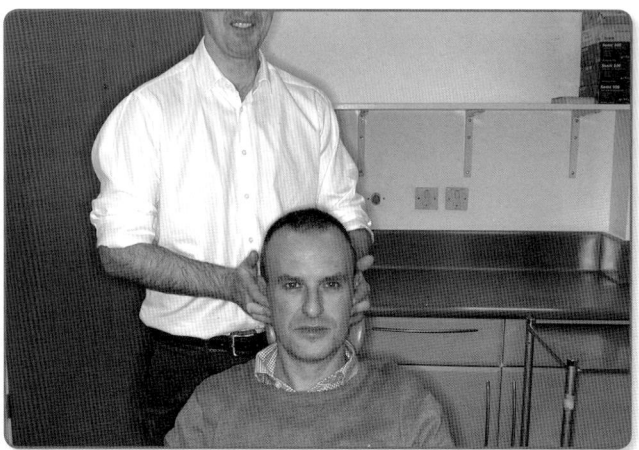

1.1 Question

How would you take a focused history in a patient presenting with TMJ problems?

Answer

- Unilateral or bilateral
- Pain: location, description (Box A) and score (1–10)
- Locking: open (dislocation) or closed (meniscal)
- Single episode or recurrent (Box B)
- Precipitating factors
- Dietary intake
- Quality of life (QoL)
- Previous or current treatments, both surgical and nonsurgical
- Frequency and duration of symptoms and aggravating/relieving factors
- Mouth opening
- Headaches
- Childhood infections
- Previous facial trauma
- Try to broadly group and classify the disorder (Boxes C and D)

1.2 Question

What conditions related to the TMJ are commonly encountered?

Answer
- TMJ total joint replacement (TJR) follow-up
- Osteochondroma
- Condylar hyperplasia
- Recurrent dislocation
- Anterior disc displacement with/without reduction (ADDwR/ADDwoR)
- Ankylosis
- Inflammatory/osteoarthritis
- Myofascial pain-predominant TMD
- Atypical facial pain (AFP)

1.3 **Question**

What associations should be explored in TMJ dysfunction?

Answer
- Stress and parafunctional habits
- Psychosocial factors
- Mental health issues (e.g. depression, anxiety)
- Headaches
- Chronic back pain
- Irritable bowel syndrome
- Fibromyalgia

1.4 **Question**

What are the factors that should be explored when taking a history in a patient with suspected ankylosis?

Answer
- Potential aetiological factors: childhood infection (especially otitis media) or trauma (e.g. intracapsular condylar fracture)
- Congenital ankylosis
- Previous surgical treatment: failed gap arthroplasty, interpositional autogenous tissue/synthetic spacers, previous distraction osteogenesis

1.5 **Question**

What are the factors that should be explored when taking a history in a patient being considered for TMJ replacement?

Answer
- Previous treatments and surgeries
- Identify how long joint has been in place
- Complications of surgery (e.g. facial weakness as graded by House-Brackmann)
- Identify indications for replacement (see 2008 guidelines paper by Sidebottom)
- Explore masticatory function, dietary intake and pain frequency and intensity

- Ask patient to compare (if possible) with their preoperative state
- Further information on outcomes measurement found in the British Association of TMJ Surgeons (BATS) 1-year outcomes paper

---

Box A: Causes of facial pain

- Remember not all facial pain is TMD
- Pain may also be odontogenic, sinusitis, neuralgia (trigeminal, postherpetic), cluster headaches, migraines, polymyalgia rheumatic (PMR)
- Sinister causes include skull base malignancy
- AFP is a diagnosis of exclusion

Box B: Recurrent dislocation

- TMJ dislocation has a number of aetiologies including excessive mouth opening, trauma, connective tissue disorders, as well as psychogenic causes
- Recurrent dislocation is often seen in the elderly with dystonia from various causes including previous stroke, dementia and neuroleptic medications
- A number of treatment strategies exist including simply teaching the patient or carer to relocate the jaw, intra-articular injection of autologous blood, exogenous sclerosants or prolotherapy, intramuscular botulinum toxin to the lateral pterygoid muscles and surgical solutions such as articular eminectomy/eminoplasty

---

Box C: Broad categorisations of TMD

- TMD may be broadly categorised as intra-articular or extra-articular
- In the former category problems relate to the articular disc, disc attachments, synovium and/or articular fibro-cartilage
- In the latter group, conditions can be musculoskeletal relating to the bone and/or masticatory muscles, and rarely, the central/peripheral nervous system
- Aim to differentiate masticatory muscle disorders from TMJ disorders, as the treatment pathways for both are very different
- Bear in mind that patients may have a combination of problems

---

Box D: Classification of TMD

- American Society of Temporomandibular Joint Surgeons Guidelines (2003)
- RDC/TMD Consortium Network criteria by Schiffman et al. (2014)

Further reading

Schiffman E, Ohrbach R, Truelove E, et al. Diagnostic criteria for temporomandibular disorders (DC/TMD) for clinical and research applications. J Oral Facial Pain Headache 2014; 28:6–27.

Short case 2: Temperomandibular joint examination

This patient presnts to clinic with recurrent painful clicking from her jaw joints.

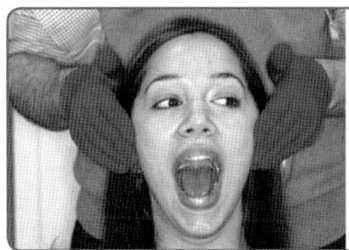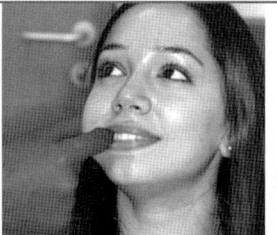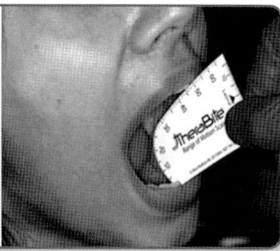

2.1 Question

What are the key points on initial inspection when examining a patient with TMJ problems as demonstrated in the figure?

Answer

- Positioning: seat the patient with Frankfort plane parallel to the floor
- Scars: access incisions for previous open arthroplasty and/or arthroscopic surgery (Box A)
- Facial asymmetry: effusion, masseteric hypertrophy
- Swelling over the joints
- Characterise the skeletal profile
- Occlusal collapse from condylar resorption with high angle anterior open bite (AOB)

2.2 Question

How would you examine the joint?

Answer

- Palpation: over lateral pole of condyle for any pain or tenderness
- Palpation: on opening or closing for any crepitus (crunching) or clicks and define when these occur
- Note any restriction to opening and establish whether due to pain or mechanical restriction
- Note any deviation or displacement

2.3 Question

What device can be used to determine mouth opening and how should it be recorded?

Answer

- The TheraBite tool is widely accepted in the UK for this purpose, particularly when ascertaining ankylosis (Box B)

- The curved side is used to measure maximum mouth opening (MMO) (>35 mm)
- The straight edge is used to measure lateral (>7 mm) and protrusive excursions
• Measure active opening and passive stretch

2.4 Question
How would you palpate the masticatory muscles?

Answer

- The masseter on opening and clenching looking for trigger points
- The temporalis muscle with the teeth clenched and muscle active
- The medial pterygoid bimanually (one finger externally at medial aspect of the angle and the other finger in the lingual vestibule intraorally)
- The lateral pterygoid intraorally posterior to the maxillary tuberosity

2.5 Question
How is the intraoral examination performed?

Answer

- Look for signs of bruxism and nocturnal clenching/grinding
- Occlusal surface wear, scalloping of tongue, pronounced linea alba and damaged restorations

2.6 Question
How would you complete the examination?

Answer

- Cranial nerve examination: facial nerve injury from previous surgery
- Evidence of systemic arthritides: peripheral joint swelling, ulnar deviation
- Auscultation of the joint with a stethoscope
- External auditor canal otoscopy
- Consider local anaesthetic injection into joint or muscle trigger points as a diagnostic aid

---

Box A: Surgical approaches to the TMJ

- The standard approaches used are the Al Kayat-Bramley approach for the fossa component and the Risdon or 'high' Risdon for the ramus component
- The former may be modified in a number of ways: endaural approach with incision carried into external auditory meatus postauricular approach dividing auditory canal

> **Box B: Causes of trismus**
> - Distinguish causes during the examination as intra-articular or extra-articular
> - The former include cause such as internal joint derangement, septic arthritis, degenerative joint changes from osteo- or inflammatory arthritis and TMJ ankylosis
> - The latter group include fibrosis of the soft tissues (e.g. radiation, submucous fibrosis, systemic sclerosis), heterotopic bone formation, local malignancy and drug-associated dystonia

Further reading

Meyer RA. The temporomandibular joint examination. In: Walter HK, Hurst JW (Eds) Clinical Methods: The History, Physical and Laboratory Examinations, 3rd Edition. Butterworths, Boston 1990.

Short case 3: Osteoarthritis (OA) of the TMJ

A patient attends your clinic with this radiograph.

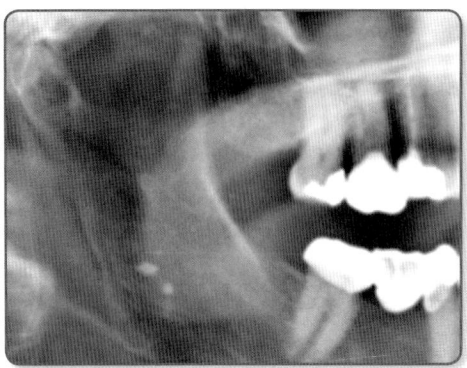

3.1 **Question**

What are the key findings in the image shown?

Answer

- Loss of joint space
- Subchondral sclerosis
- Subchondral cyst formation

3.2 **Question**

What is the likely diagnosis and are there any other radiological features that you would expect which are not shown in the Figure?

Answer

- TMJ osteoarthritis
- Classical radiological signs are listed in Box A

3.3 **Question**

What are the key features in the history?

Answer

- Dietary score
- Pain score
- Quality of life
- Progression of symptoms
- Previous nonsurgical treatment
- Previous surgical interventions
- Co-existing joint problems elsewhere and/or diagnosed arthritides

3.4 Question

What are the most likely examination findings?

Answer

- Maximum mouth opening (MMO) measured by interincisal distance
- Lateral and protrusive excursions
- Pain and/or crepitus/clicks over TMJ
- Associated (secondary) myofascial pain
- Other features of systemic arthritides, e.g. psoriatic plaques, peripheral joint involvement

3.5 Question

What further investigations might be required?

Answer

- Arthroscopy and cross-sectional imaging are strongly advised if considering eventual joint replacement
- Computed tomography (CT) should be performed as delineating bony anatomy
- CT will facilitate custom alloplastic replacement, e.g. ProtoMED protocol for TMJ concepts devices

3.6 Question

What are the treatment options?

Answer

- Early management strategies may include topical NSAIDs, avoiding precipitants, TMJ physiotherapy and analgesia
- Intra-articular steroid injection with or without arthrocentesis or arthroscopy may give symptomatic benefit and dampen the inflammatory response (Box B)
- Arthroscopy may also be diagnostic and a precursor of more invasive treatment

3.7 Question

When should open surgery be considered and what are the main surgical options?

Answer

- When conservative and minimally invasive options have failed
- Arthroplasty and joint replacement (Box C)

3.8 Question

How is arthroplasty performed?

Answer

- Typically, an Al-Khayat-Bramley approach is used
- Remove all osteophytes
- Repair meniscal tears
- Remove unsalvageable discs
- Reshape condylar head

Box A: Radiographic features of OA

- Nonuniform joint space loss
- Osteophyte formation
- Cyst formation
- Subchondral sclerosis

Box B: Steroids in TMJ OA

- Intra-articular steroid injection (IASI) may be considered for OA that has been unresponsive to conservative measures in order to reduce pain and improve function. This may be done in isolation or as part of arthrocentesis/arthroscopy
- There is evidence to suggest that IASI is superior to placebo
- A recent meta-analysis by Liu and colleagues (2017) highlighted that hyaluronate may be preferential to corticosteroid in terms of improved MMO as an outcome measure. osteoarthritis (OA)

Box C: Joint replacement

- This is best regarded as a last resort and indications for joint replacement have been set out in the 2008 paper by Andrew Sidebottom on behalf of UK TMJ surgeons and comprises
- Diet score <5/10
- MMO <35 mm
- Occlusal collapse
- Excessive condylar resorption/loss of height
- Pain score >5/10

Further reading

Dimitroulis G. The role of surgery in the management of disorders of the temporomandibular joint: a critical review of the literature Part 2. Int J Oral Maxillofac Surg 2005; 34:231–237.

Liu Y, Wu J, Fei W, et al. Is there a difference in intra-articular injections of corticosteroids, hyaluronate or placebo for temporomandibular osteoarthritis? J Oral Maxillofac Surg 2017; 76:504–514.

Rajapakse S, Ahmed N, Sidebottom AJ. Current thinking about the management of dysfunction of the temporomandibular joint: a review. Br J Oral Maxillofac Surg 2017; 55:351–356.

Short case 4: Synovial chondromatosis and MRI

This patient presents with unilateral TMJ pain with recent imaging shown in the figure.

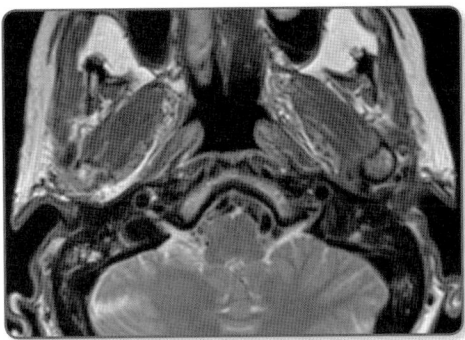

4.1 Question
What is the likely spot diagnosis and the underlying cause?

Answer
- Likely represents synovial chondromatosis (Box A)
- Cause is idiopathic (Box B)

4.2 Question
What are the key features when taking a history in a patient as described above?

Answer
- Symptoms may include: pain, swelling, trismus, clicking/crepitus of affected joint, malocclusion
- Advanced stages may include: vertigo; tinnitus; cranial nerve dysfunction

4.3 Question
What are the key examination features?

Answer
- Unilateral preauricular swelling/pain
- Deviations/displacements on opening/closing
- Clicking/crepitus
- Palpable foreign bodied in advanced cases
- Arthroscopy/arthroplasty scar(s), e.g. Al Khayat-Bramley incision
- Maximum mouth opening

4.4 Question

What investigations would you propose?

Answer

- Cross-sectional imaging, e.g. CT/MRI
- Arthroscopy and/or specimen for histology (Box C)

4.5 Question

What are the key radiographic features?

Answer

- Features may include widening of joint space, sclerosis, flattening of articular surfaces, hyperplasia, erosion of both fossa and condyle
- Calcified loose bodies are only seen in 30% of plain film radiographs and 53% of CTs
- MRI may demonstrate swelling in lateral capsule and joint effusion. In extreme cases there may be destruction of skull base

4.6 Question

What are the treatment options?

Answer

- Arthroscopic removal of loose bodies with coagulation of synovium with bipolar electrocautery/radiofrequency
- Open arthroplasty to remove loose bodies, particularly if exhibiting extracapsular extension and/or loose bodies >3 mm
- May require removal of affected synovium (synovectomy) and/or condylectomy and/or discectomy

4.7 Question

What is the risk of malignant change?

Answer

- A 5% risk has historically been described in large joints but this is now considered to be an over-estimate
- Only three case reports exist of malignant change occurring in TMJ (chondrosarcoma)
- May be an association with pigmented villonodular synovitis

---

Box A: Synovial chondromatosis

- Rare pathologic condition characterized by formation of metaplastic cartilaginous nodules in the synovium and articular space
- Two forms recognized: primary (idiopathic) and secondary (e.g. following trauma)

> **Box B: Aetiology**
> - Unknown in the primary form but three stages proposed
> - Metaplasia of synovial membrane
> - Progressive metaplasia causing detachment of loose bodies
> - Loose bodies containing chondrocytes degenerate and calcify
> - More commonly involves upper joint space (some postulate exclusively)
> - Mean age of presentation 4th and 5th decades
> - Females affected more commonly than males
> - Peripheral joint involvement, e.g. prosthetic joints, scars of previous arthroscopy

> **Box C: Histology of synovial chondromatosis**
> - Benign chronic inflammation of synovium (synovitis) with metaplastic activity with three stages described by Milgram (1977)
> - Active intrasynovial disease with no loose bodies
> - Transitional lesions with intrasynovial proliferation and loose bodies
> - Multiple free osteochondral bodies
> - Degeneration is seen in the synovial membrane (myxoid) and cartilage (cystic degeneration)

Further reading

Hodder SC, Rees JI, Oliver TB, et al. SPECT bone scintigraphy in the diagnosis and management of mandibular condylar hyperplasia. Br J Oral Maxillofac Surg 2000; 38:87–93.

Nitzan DW, Katsnelson A, Bermanis I, et al. The clinical characteristics of condylar hyperplasia: experience with 61 patients. J Oral Maxillofac Surg 2008; 66:312–318.

Obwegeser HL, Makek HS. Hemimandibular hyperplasia – hemimandibular elongation. J Maxillofac Surg 1986; 14:183–208.

Wolford LM, Mehra P, Reiche-Fischel O, et al. Efficacy of high condylectomy for management of condylar hyperplasia. Am J Orthod Dentofacial Orthop 2002; 121:136–150.

Short case 5: Closed lock and MRI

This patient returns to clinic having previously complained of repeated bouts of locking of the jaw.

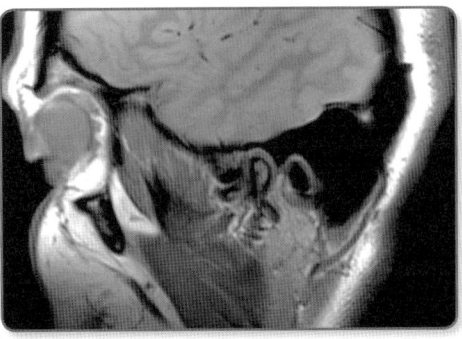

5.1 Question

Based upon the image shown, what are the key features in the history?

Answer

- Clarify exacerbating and relieving factors
- Ask about frequency of locking and trismus
- Any previous surgery/arthroscopy/arthrocentesis
- Associated pain and headaches

5.2 Question

The jaw locks when their teeth are almost closed and they cannot open further. What is the likely diagnosis?

Answer

- ADDWOR
- Articular disc is malpositioned (Box A)

5.3 Question

What are the key features that are likely to be demonstrated on examination?

Answer

- Unilateral preauricular swelling/pain
- Deviations/displacements on opening/closing
- Establish whether the patient can 'manoeuvre' their jaw to achieve maximal opening (i.e. overcome the anterior disc displacement to 'recapture' the disc)
- Clicking/crepitus
- Maximum mouth opening

5.4 Question

What is the value of requesting an MR?

Answer

- MR correlates well with clinical signs and symptoms – in particular joint effusion and marrow oedema correlating with pain
- MRI showed a specificity of 84% and sensitivity of 73% for ADDWOR in one study

5.5 Question

What are the key radiographic features?

Answer

- ADDWOR (Box B)
- Moderate to marked disc thickening

5.6 Question

How would you manage the patient further?

Answer

- Attempt to classify in order to help guide treatment (Box C)
- All patients should initially be managed with a conservative regim
- Rest, NSAIDs, bite splint, avoidance of precipitating factors and self-directed TMJ exercises for at least 6 weeks

5.7 Question

What are the options if conservative treatment fails?

Answer

- Arthrocentesis or arthroscopy are both valid options and the decision between the two is very clinician dependent
- Both have similar response rates (>80%, Box D)
- Arthroscopy yields greater diagnostic information, but with increased risk of complications

5.8 Question

What are the potential complications of arthroscopy?

Answer

- Complication rate reported as ranging from 1.8% to 10.3%
- Facial nerve injury
- Trigeminal nerve deficit
- Otic injury
- Preauricular haematoma
- Superficial temporal artery aneurysm

- Arteriovenous fistula
- Transarticular perforation
- Intracranial perforation
- Extradural haematoma
- Parapharyngeal swelling and intra-articular swelling

Box A: The articular disc and potential displacement

- The articular disc is a firm, fibrocartilaginous structure with a biconcave shape
- It has three regions: central zone (1 mm), posterior zone (3 mm), anterior zone (2 mm)
- Posteriorly it is contiguous with posterior attachment tissues (bilaminar zone, retrodiscal laminae) adhering to the temporal bone and neck of condyle
- Anteriorly, the disc, capsule and fascia of the superior head of lateral pterygoid are contiguous
- TMJ disc displacement is a disorder characterized by the abnormal position of the articular disc in relation to the mandibular condyle and the mandibular fossa

---

Box B: Radiological features of ADDWR

- Position, morphology, signal intensity and structure of the articular disc
- Quantity of synovial fluid, effusions
- Condition of the posterior attachment and retrodiscal tissues, presence/absence of disc deformity
- Marrow oedema

Box C: The Wilkes system

- The Wilkes system classifies internal joint derangement based on clinical, radiographic and surgical findings as stages I–V
- Locking, frequent pain and restricted motion are clinical features of stage III

Box D: Arthrocentesis

- A number of different techniques of arthrocentesis have been described
- These include two-needle techniques, the double-needle cannula (Shepard cannula), single-needle arthrocentesis and a variety of landmarks
- Various authors have described instilling morphine, bupivacaine, fentanyl, methylprednisolone, triamcinolone and sodium hyaluronate among other agents
- Recommended amounts of irrigant also vary, with many postulating that it is the initial hydrodissection prior to introducing the second needle that has the greatest therapeutic benefit

Further reading

Ahmed N, Sidebottom A, O'Connor M, Kerr HL. Prospective outcome assessment of the therapeutic benefits of arthroscopy and arthrocentesis of the temporomandibular joint. Br J Oral Maxillofac Surg 2012; 50:745–748.

Tozoglu S, Al-Belasy FA, Franklin Dolwick M. A review of techniques of lysis and lavage of the TMJ. Br J Oral Maxillofac Surg 2011; 49:302–309.

Vogl TJ, Lauer JC, Lehnert T, et al. The value of MRI in patients with temporomandibular joint dysfunction: correlation of MRI and clinical findings. Eur J Radiol 2016; 85:714–719.

Wilkes CH. Internal derangements of the temporomandibular joint. Pathological variations. Northwest Dent 1990; 69:25–32.

Short case 6: SPECT interpretation

The patient shown in the figure returns to clinic.

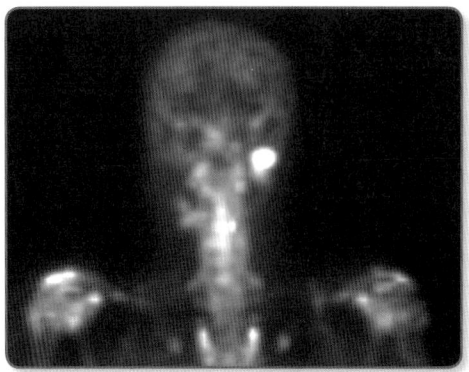

6.1 **Question**

What are the key features in the history to ask about?

Answer

- Progressive asymmetry of face noted by patients or others
- Swelling and/or pain around condyle
- Accompanying symptoms of myofascial pain
- Diet score, pain score, quality of life

6.2 **Question**

What are the key examination features?

Answer

- Preauricular swelling/pain
- Deviations/displacements on opening/closing
- Crossbite
- Dental midline shift
- Chin point displacement
- Lateral open bite
- Maxillary cant

6.3 **Question**

What investigations would you propose?

Answer

- Study models
- Plain films: OPG/lateral cephalogram
- Photographs: progression
- SPECT: condylar activity (Box A)

6.4 Question

What potential conditions may present with swelling of the condylar area?

Answer
- Condylar hyperplasia (Box B)
- Osteochondroma (Box C)

6.5 Question

What is the key finding on the SPECT scan to indicate condylar hyperplasia?

Answer
- Relative uptake increase of 55% or more in the affected condyle as described by Hodder et al.

6.6 Question

What are the treatment options?

Answer
- Allow condylar hyperplasia to 'burn out' then follow with conventional orthognathic surgery to manage residual deformity
- High condylar shave with serial SPECT and/or study models to assess stability and then orthognathic surgery to manage residual deformity
- 'Wolford et al.' described condylectomy in conjunction with articular disc repositioning (meniscopexy) but this is generally not recommended

6.7 Question

How are osteochondromas managed?

Answer
- Complete condylectomy and autogenous/alloplastic TMJ reconstruction
- Orthognathic correction of deformity performed secondarily
- Wolford et al. described a more conservative 'low condylectomy' and ramus height preservation, recontouring the condylar neck
- Other options: condylectomy and vertical osteotomy of the ramus to advance superiorly as a surrogate condyle

---

Box A: Single Photon Emission Computer Tomography
- Useful for differentiating metabolic activity between condyles
- Role in the diagnosis of condylar hyperplasia (CH) or osteochondroma
- Be wary of false positives, e.g. inflammation, infection, post-traumatic

> **Box B: Condylar hyperplasia**
> - Best thought of as three distinct entities as per Obwegeser and Makek
> - Hemimandibular hyperplasia (HH) in which the entire hemimandible is enlarged, the chin point is apparent ipsilateral and the centerline is preserved
> - Hemimandibular elongation (HE) in which the condylar neck is lengthened and the chin point is contralateral with a centerline shift
> - A combination of HH and HE

> **Box C: Osteochondromas**
> - Rare, slow-growing benign neoplasm of the condylar head
> - Radiographically presents as unilateral, enlarged, deformed condyle and associated dentofacial deformity
> - Clinically presents as malocclusion, lateral open bite, dental and chin-point shift, occlusal cant and progressive facial asymmetry

Further reading

Hodder SC, Rees JI, Oliver TB, et al. SPECT bone scintigraphy in the diagnosis and management of mandibular condylar hyperplasia. Br J Oral Maxillofac Surg 2000; 38:87–93.

Nitzan DW, Katsnelson A, Bermanis I, et al. The clinical characteristics of condylar hyperplasia: experience with 61 patients. J Oral Maxillofac Surg 2008; 66:312–318.

Obwegeser HL, Makek HS. Hemimandibular hyperplasia – hemimandibular elongation. J Maxillofac Surg 1986; 14:183–208.

Wolford LM, Mehra P, Reiche-Fischel O, et al. Efficacy of high condylectomy for management of condylar hyperplasia. Am J Orthod Dentofacial Orthop 2002; 121:136–150.

Short case 7: Alloplastic TMJ replacement

Prior to surgery you sit down with your specialist trainee to discuss the critical steps.

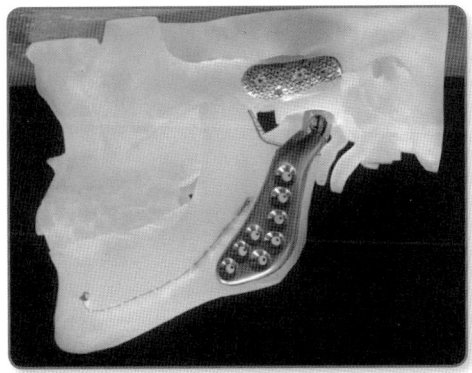

7.1 Question

In this figure, what procedure is the patient being planned for and what are the components of the prosthesis?

Answer

- Alloplastic total joint replacement
- Prosthesis comprises of two components: the condylar head and fossa (Box A)
- Head is made of titanium with cobalt-chromium alloy and fixes to the osteotomised ramus
- Fossa component is made of high-molecular weight polyethylene and screws directly over the existing fossa (Box B)

7.2 Question

What are the key features to identify when examining this patient in clinic?

Answer

- Scars: including Al Kayat-Bramley and Risdon approaches
- Maximum mouth opening
- Protrusive and lateral excursions
- Deviation towards prosthesis (this is normal)
- Any dislocation of prosthesis
- Any associated myofascial pain

7.3 Question

What is the work-up for a TJR?

Answer
- Allergy testing: chrome, cobalt, molybdenum or nickel mandate all-titanium devices
- CT: specific protocols are usually required when the scan is performed to optimise prosthesis fabrication

7.4 Question
What are the indications for considering a TJR?

Answer
- Dietary score <5/10
- MMO <35 mm
- Pain score >5/10
- Excessive condylar resorption
- Diseases treated may include osteoarthritis, inflammatory arthritides, ankylosis, trauma, previous failed reconstruction and severe congenital deformity
- Failed conservative management (Box C)

7.5 Question
The patient asks what the lifespan is. What will you tell them?

Answer
- Long-term outcomes do not currently exist (Box D)
- Wolford et al. (2015) published a 20-year follow-up of TMJ Concepts devices demonstrating sustained improvements in QoL in 48/56 patients

7.6 Question
What national guidance exists?

Answer
- NICE guidelines (2014): total prosthetic replacement of the temporomandibular joint. These guidelines provide indications and reports on cross-sectional data from 425 patients noting a device failure rate of 19/215 (9%) where data was available

7.7 Question
What is an extended TMJ replacement (TJRE) and what are the indications for one?

Answer
- TJRE additionally address segmental mandibular deficiencies and/or base of skull deficiencies due to congenital or acquired causes
  TJRE devices have extensions of both ramus and/or fossa components
- Indications include Goldenhar syndrome, SAPHO syndrome, hemifacial microsomia (HFM), and ablative oncological resections

Box A: Components of prostheses

- Early devices included the stainless steel fossa prosthesis (Robinson, 1960) and vitallium fossae (Christensen)
- Proplast (polytetrafluoroethylene) was used as a laminant in the VK system, but demonstrated foreign body reactions from particulate debris
- Delrin (polyoxymethylene) was tried but caused heterotopic bone formation
- Modern devices use metal (titanium with cobalt-chromium alloy) ramus on high-molecular weight polyethylene in the fossa

Box B: Identifying TMJ TJRs

- There are a wide variety of total alloplastic TMJ TJRs in use around the world
- In the UK, Speculand's 2009 paper on the history of TMJ TJR is a good reference point for any devices likely to be encountered
- The two companies currently providing devices currently used in the UK are TMJ Concepts (Ventura, CA) and Zimmer Biomet (Jacksonville, FL)
- It is advisable to be familiar with the radiographic and clinical appearance of both
- Extended TMJ replacement devices are less likely to be seen but a recently published classification system exists

Box C: Prerequisites for TJR

- Patients should have as a minimum failed conservative management (including arthroscopy where possible) and have cross-sectional imaging available (CT/MRI)
- There should be no local infection or severe immunocompromise, and in particular patients should have otoscopy on the day of the procedure. TJR should be postponed in the presence of active ear infection
- Finally, disease-modifying anti-rheumatic drugs (DMARDs) should be stopped

Box D: UK TMJ replacement outcomes

- In the UK outcomes reporting for TMJ replacements is in its infancy with a one-year outcomes paper published
- Wolford et al. (2015) reporting outcomes beyond 20 years for TMJ Concepts devices

Further reading

Elledge R, Attard A, Green J, et al. UK temporomandibular joint replacement database: a report on one-year outcomes. Br J Oral Maxillofac Surg 2017; 55:927–931.

Elledge R, Mercuri LG, Speculand B. Extended total temporomandibular joint replacements: a classification system. Br J Oral Maxillofac Surg 2018; 56:578–581.

Elledge R, Attard A, Green J, et al. UK temporomandibular joint replacement database: a report on one-year outcomes. Br J Oral Maxillofac Surg 2017; 55:927–931.

National Institute for Health and Clinical Excellence. Total prosthetic replacement of the temporomandibular joint. Interventional procedures guidance [IPG500]. August 2014.

Sidebottom AJ. Guidelines for the replacement of temporomandibular joints in the United Kingdom. Br J Oral Maxillofac Surg 2008; 46:146–147.

Speculand B. Current status of replacement of the temporomandibular joint in the United Kingdom. Br J Oral Maxillofac Surg 2009; 47:37–41.

Short case 8: Recurrent TMJ dislocation

A patient with this radiograph presents with their carer complaining of difficulty in eating.

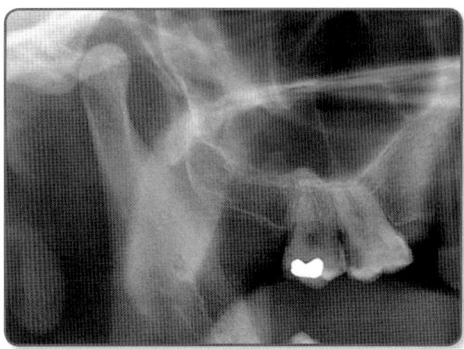

8.1 Question
What is the likely diagnosis?

Answer

- The patient has TMJ dislocation without reduction. The radiograph shows the right condylar head lying anterior to the articular eminence

8.2 Question
This is their second presentation of TMJ dislocation. What are the key points in the history?

Answer

- Frequency of dislocation
- Duration
- Precipitating events: yawning, vomiting, seizures
- Ability to 'self-reduce' (patient or carer)
- Medical co-morbidities: neurological conditions, connective tissue disorders, neuroleptic medications (as potential causes of dystonia)
- Psycho-social overlay (Box A)

8.3 Question
What are the key points in the examination?

Answer

- Range of opening
- Displacements/deviations
- Clicks and/or crepitus

- Spontaneous dislocation and/or apprehension on protrusive and lateral excursions, quantifying the limits of these movements

8.4 Question

What are the nonsurgical treatment options for recurrent TMJ dislocation?

Answer

- Medications: muscle relaxants, antispasmodics
- Psychological management
- Physical therapy
- Intermaxillary fixation
- Injection of sclerosing agent injection, including autologous blood (Box B)
- Botulinum toxin injection: to lateral pterygoid muscles

8.5 Question

What are the surgical options?

Answer

- Soft tissue procedures
- Eminectomy
- Creation of a mechanical obstacle: Dautrey/LeClerc procedure (Box C)
- Tethering techniques
- Mandibular osteotomies: condylotomy/condylectomy

8.6 Question

What are the options for restricting joint movement surgically?

Answer

- Lateral pterygoid myotomy, capsular plication and scarification of temporalis muscle are all options for restricting joint movement
- TMJ ligament and bilaminar tissue scarification may be done arthroscopically, e.g. using the holmium Nd:YAG laser
- Ligamentorrhaphy may be performed by fixing the lateral capsule to the zygomatic arch
- Mitek anchors have also been used with sutures acting to restrain lateral pole of condyle
- Temporalis fascia may also be used in this way

8.7 Question

How does eminectomy work?

Answer

- Used to enable 'free' movement of the condyle
- Requires bone removal to a depth of at least 2 cm
- Small but significant risk of intracranial perforation in inexperienced hands

Box A: Mental health and recurrent dislocation

- The interplay here is complex
- Many antipsychotic medications may cause dystonia, rendering TMJ dislocation more likely
- In addition, orofacial pain in general and TMJ disorders are more common in patients with eating disorders, particularly bulimia
- There are documented instances of self-induced recurrent dislocation as part of attention-seeking or Munchausen syndrome, characterized by 'peregrination' (multiple visits to different hospitals for the same simulated illness)

Box B: Prolotherapy and sclerosants

- Autologous blood injections have been well established for the treatment of recurrent TMJ dislocation
- Machon et al. (2009) described using 3 mL, with 2 mL being injected into the upper joint space and 1 mL into the pericapsular tissues
- A wide variety of exogenous sclerosants have also been used including ethanolamine oleate, 100% ethanol, bleomycin, OK-432, sodium tetradecyl sulphate (STS)
- 'Prolotherapy' is the intra-articular injection of nonsclerosants to initiate an inflammatory response, e.g. hypertonic (10–50%) dextrose

Box C: The Dautrey/LeClerc procedure

- Down-fracturing of a portion of the zygomatic arch to prevent anterior translation of the condylar head
- Advantages purported were preservation of the joint (the procedure is extracapsular) and little or no trismus
- High success rates have been reported
- Generally felt to be outmoded and principally of historical interest

Further reading

Elledge R, Speculand B. Conservative management options for dislocation of the temporomandibular joint. In: Matthews NS (Ed) Dislocation of the Temporomandibular Joint. Springer International Publishing, 2018.

Machon V, Abramowicz S, Paska J, Dolwick MF. Autologous blood injection for the treatment of recurrent temporomandibular joint dislocation. J Oral Maxillofac Surg 2009; 67:114–119.

Sarlabous M, Psutka DJ. Surgical management: obstructing the path. In: Matthews NS (Ed) Dislocation of the Temporomandibular Joint. Springer International Publishing, 2018.

Long case 9: TMJ ankylosis

The patient with this CT image has been referred to your clinic.

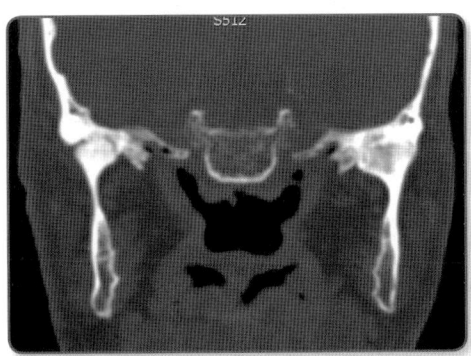

9.1 Question
What is the spot diagnosis?

Answer
- Bilateral TMJ ankylosis (Box A)
- Complete obliteration of joint space on left joint, and to a lesser degree on right side
- Left side could be classified as type 4 using the classification described by Sawhney (Box B)

9.2 Question
What are the key features in the history?

Answer
- Absolute trismus
- Progression
- Diet, weight loss, dental health (difficulty brushing teeth)
- Preceding risk factors, e.g. history of trauma (condylar fractures), middle ear infections
- Inflammatory arthropathies, e.g. rheumatoid, psoriatic

9.3 Question
What are the key examination features?

Answer
- Maximum mouth opening (which may be effectively 0 mm)
- Protrusive/lateral excursions
- Bony swelling over condyles
- Calcification of muscles of mastication (myositis ossificans)

9.4 Question

What investigations would you use to determine your management plan?

Answer

- Orthopantomogram (panorex)
- Computer tomography (CT) with 3D reformatting and/or model printing
- Angiography and/or embolisation due to proximity of internal maxillary artery and pterygoid plexus has been advocated

9.5 Question

What are the treatment options for treating TMJ ankylosis?

Answer

Surgical excision of ankylotic mass followed by replacement with:
- Interpositional autogenous graft, e.g. temporalis, abdominal fat
- Temporary silicone spacer with a view to planning delayed reconstruction with prosthetic TMJ replacement
- Immediate reconstruction with autogenous graft, e.g. costochondral graft (CCG)
- One stage replacement with alloplastic TMJ replacement

9.6 Question

What is the treatment of choice in children?

Answer

- The seven-step so-called Kaban protocol is often used (Box C)
- Aggressive excision
- Ipsilateral and/or contralateral coronoidectomy
- CCG or distraction osteogenesis (DO)
- Aggressive physiotherapy with early mobilisation

9.7 Question

Which device can be used to achieve early mobilisation?

Answer

- Best achieved with a TheraBite Jaw Motion Rehabilitation System

9.8 Question

What is a potential problem of CCG reconstruction in children?

Answer

- Unpredictability of growth
- One-third undergrow, one-third overgrow and the remainder keep pace with the child's growth; however, a recent systematic review by Kumar et al. has questioned this theory

Box A: Definition of ankylosis

- Fusion of the condyle with the skull base
- Important to distinguish that fusion may be fibrous, fibro-osseous or bone, complete or incomplete
- Common aetiologies include otitis media, mastoiditis, haematogenous spread from diseases, e.g. tuberculosis, gonorrhea, ankylosing spondylitis, rheumatoid arthritis, psoriatic arthritis

Box B: Classification of ankylosis

- A number of different severity classification systems exist
- Topazian (1966) classified based on extent of ankylotic bone mass
- Sawhney (1986) classification is given as follows:
  - Type I: fibrous adhesions around joint
  - Type II: bony fusion at lateral articular surface
  - Type III: bony bridge between ascending ramus of mandible and temporal bone/zygomatic arch
  - Type IV: joint replaced by mass of bone between ramus and skull base

Box C: The 'Kaban protocol'

- Aggressive excision of fibrous/bony mass
- Coronoidectomy affected side
- Coronoidectomy contralateral side if MMO <35 mm
- Lining of joint with temporalis myofascial flap (or disc salvage)
- Reconstruction with CCG or DO
- Early mobilisation of jaw
- Aggressive physiotherapy

Further reading

Arakeri G, Kusanale A, Zaki GA, Brennan PA. Pathogenesis of post-traumatic ankylosis of the temporomandibular joint: a critical review. Br J Oral Maxillofac Surg 2012; 50:8–12.

Kaban LB, Bouchard C, Troulis MJ. A protocol for management of temporomandibular joint ankylosis in children. J Oral Maxillofac Surg 2009; 67:1966–1978.

Kumar P, Rattan V, Rai S. Do costochondral grafts have any growth potential in temporomandibular joint surgery? A systematic review. J Oral Biol Craniofac Res 2015; 5:198–202.

Sawhney CP. Bony ankylosis of the temporomandibular joint: follow-up of 70 patients treated with arthroplasty and acrylic spacer interposition. Plast Reconstr Surg 1986; 77:29–40.

Chapter 9

Craniofacial and paediatric surgery

SHORT CASES

1. Assessment of the craniofacial and syndromic child
2. Distraction osteogenesis
3. Temporal hollowing
4. LeFort III advancement
5. Zygomaticus implants

LONG CASE

6. Arteriovenous vascular malformation

Short case 1: Assessment of the craniofacial and syndromic child

A general practitioner has referred the baby shown in the figure to your craniofacial clinic with concerns about their head shape.

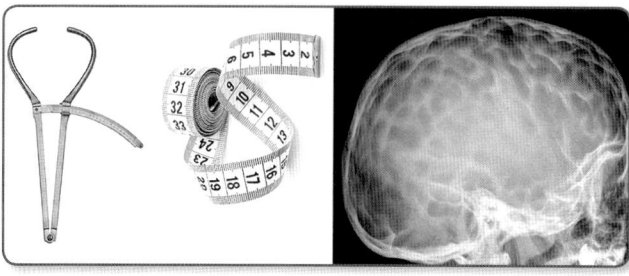

1.1 Question

What are the key points in the history?

Answer

- Age at referral (Box A)
- Parental details: age, consanguinity, family history of abnormality
- Referral source: GP, emergency department, paediatrician, secondary care
- Presenting complaint: most commonly altered head shape or developmental delay
- Prenatal history: maternal illness and drugs
- Birth history: method of delivery, prematurity
- Symptoms of raised intracranial pressure (Box B)
- Developmental milestones: delay is a late sign
- Red book: assessment of growth charts
- Performance at school or playgroup
- Medical and drug history

1.2 Question

Using the plastic skull with the instruments above show how you would you examine the patient?

Answer

- End of the bed: general appearance and obvious syndromic features (Box C)
- Skull examination: shape, presence, size and tension of fontanelles, ridging of sutures, saddle deformity, asymmetry
- Facial examination: assess eyes/ears/mouth/nose for stigmata of syndromic condition
- Limb examination: hands and feet

Short case 1 Assessment of the craniofacial and syndromic child

1.3 Question

What additional measurements would you perform in clinic?

Answer
- Head circumference: using measuring tape
- Cephalic index: using callipers (Box D)

1.4 Question

You measure the cephalic index as 62. What can this represent?

Answer
- A cephalic index less than 70 suggests scaphocephaly (increased anteroposterior dimension)
- Scaphocephaly may be due to sagittal suture synostosis (Box C)

1.5 Question

How would you investigate potentially raised ICP?

Answer
- Raised ICP: mainly occurs in multi suture synostosis
- Ophthalmology referral: to assess for papilloedema
- CT scan: may require sedation or GA
- MRI scan: requires GA and is more effective at examining the brain
- When results equivocal, consider intracranial pressure monitoring for 48 hours

1.6 Question

There are no concerns about raised ICP but due to the head shape the mother wants further investigations. What would you do?

Answer
- Reassure the mother and review the child when 9 months old
- If the head shape is still abnormal and there is concern about potential synostosis then request CT scan

1.7 Question

You are shown the radiograph in the figure. What can you see and what may it represent?

Answer
- Skull of a child with a copper beaten appearance
- May represent raised ICP or rickets (renal or vitamin D deficiency)

1.8 Question

What are the long-term consequences of raised ICP?

Answer
- Headaches
- Intellectual disability: developmental delay
- Blindness

1.9 Question

If investigations suggest raised ICP what would you do?

Answer
- ICP monitoring: using a bolt (never lumbar puncture)
- Surgery: usually vault expansion, occasionally a shunt or an endoscopic third ventriculostomy cerebrospinal fluid diversion procedure (ETV)

Box A: Age of presentation

- At birth or early infancy with altered appearance
- Later with neurodevelopmental delay

Box B: Symptoms suggestive of raised intracranial pressure (ICP)

- Unconsolable crying
- Headaches, especially on waking or with exercise
- Irritability
- Head banging
- Poor sleep
- May be asymptomatic especially in younger children

Box C: Most commonly encountered craniofacial syndromes

- Crouzons
- Apert
- Pfeiffer
- Muenke (Pro250Arg)
- Craniofacial microsomia: implying skull involvement rather than just facial as in hemi-facial
- Saethre–Chotzen
- Treacher Collins

> **Box D: Cranial (cephalic) index**
> - Biparietal (breadth) width divided by anteroposterior (length) x 100
> - Normal ratio depends if baby lying on back or side, breech presentation, twin pregnancy
> - Normal: approximately 75
> - Brachycephaly (short AP): >80
> - Scaphocephaly: <70
> - In trigonocephaly, the cephalic index is normal, but there is bitemporal hollowing and biparietal broadening

Further reading

Taylor JA, Bartlett SP. What's New in Syndromic Craniosynostosis Surgery? Plast Reconstr Surg 2017; 140:82e–93e.

Short case 2: Distraction osteogenesis

The patient shown in this figure has come to the clinic for follow-up.

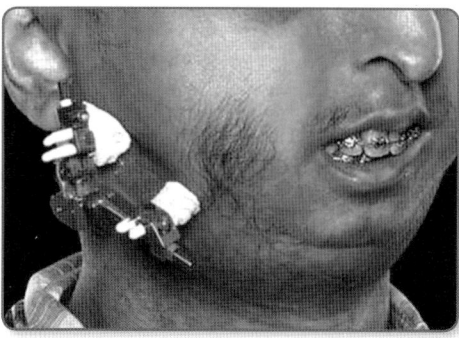

2.1 Question
Describe what you can see.

Answer
- Patient has a single vector mandibular distractor for performing distraction osteogenesis (Box A and B)

2.2 Question
What are the relevant points in the history?

Answer
- Indication for procedure: syndromic or nonsyndromic patient (Box C and D)
- Stage of distraction (Box E)
- Complications from surgery: pain, infection, TMJ discomfort

2.3 Question
What are the key points in the examination?

Answer
- End of the bed: syndromic features
- Skeletal class
- Anterior facial height
- FMP angle
- Incisal relationship
- Complications from distractor: erythema, pin site infection, loosening of pins
- TMJ: pain on palpation, mouth opening

2.4 Question

How do you know when to stop distraction?

Answer

- Preoperative plan should determine post distraction position of mandible
- In some cases, over-distraction is advantageous as this will enable a degree of relapse or account for further facial growth (particularly in younger children)
- Progress of distraction can be determined by chin position and lower incisor position, both AP and transverse (overjet and lower midline)

2.5 Question

What are the advantages of distraction over conventional osteotomy?

Answer

- Avoids requirement for bone grafts with resultant morbidity and hospital stay
- Can be performed at young age
- Enables larger skeletal movements
- Simultaneous lengthening of soft tissues

2.6 Question

What are the disadvantages of distraction over conventional osteotomy?

Answer

- External skin scars of distraction
- Pin loosening or pin site infection
- Greater patient and family compliance required
- Greater clinical supervision and outpatient follow-up required
- Marginal mandibular nerve injuries

2.7 Question

Is distraction more stable than a standard BSSO?

Answer

- No difference in long-term stability
- Lack of quality clinical trials
- Some evidence that distraction may be better for low angle patients requiring large advancements (>7 mm)

2.8 Question

What are the advantages of internal over external distraction?

Answer

- Better aesthetics when device in situ
- No scarring from fixation pins being dragged through tissues

2.9 Question

What are the disadvantages of internal devices over external?

Answer
- Placement and removal of devices may be challenging
- Greater disruption to periosteum and blood supply
- More difficult to distract large distances compared to extraoral devices
- More difficult to produce multivector movements

Box A: Broad types of distraction devices

Internal:
- Generally univector (although curvilinear internal distractors are used)
- Device almost entirely buried beneath the soft tissues
- Activation rod may lie in the buccal sulcus or exit transcutaneously

External:
- Can be uni or multivector
- Placed almost entirely outside the skin
- Multiple pins that pass transcutaneously into the bone

Box B: Commonly utilised types of vectors

- Single vector: linear or curvilinear
- Multiple vector

Box C: Potential indications for mandibular distraction

- Syndromic hypoplasia (Box D)
- Extreme nonsyndromic mandibular retrognathia
- Obstructive sleep apnoea
- Post-traumatic deformity, e.g. ballistic
- Postoncological resection

Box D: Syndromes mandibular distraction commonly used for

- Hemifacial microsomia
- Treacher Collins syndrome
- Pierre Robin sequence
- Nagar Syndrome

Box E: Principles of distraction

- Corticotomy (immediate): osteotomy separates bone cortices
- Latency (commonly 1–3 days): formation of early callus between bone ends
- Activation (commonly 0.5 mm twice daily): bone ends progressively separated
- Consolidation (number of days 3–4 times the distance moved): ossification of callus

Further reading

Baas EM, de Lange J, Horsthuis RB. Evaluation of alveolar nerve function after surgical lengthening of the mandible by a bilateral sagittal split osteotomy or distraction osteogenesis. Int J Oral Maxillofac Surg 2010; 39:529–533.

Vos MD, Baas EM, de Lange J, et al. Stability of mandibular advancement procedures: bilateral sagittal split osteotomy versus distraction osteogenesis. Int J Oral Maxillofac Surg 2009; 38:7–12.

Short case 3: Temporal hollowing

The patient shown in the figure sustained facial trauma 1 year ago and now dislikes the appearance of her temple.

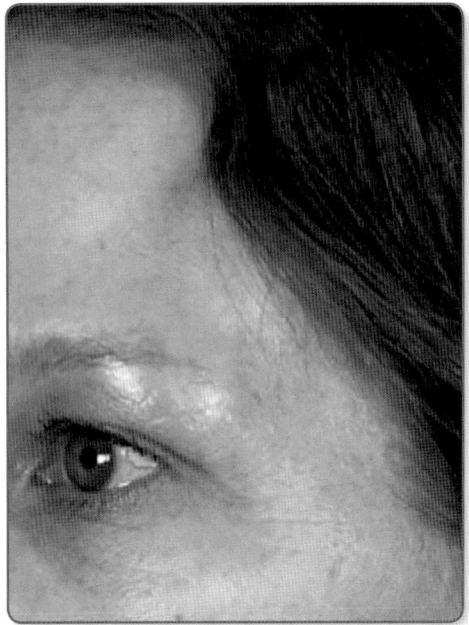

3.1 Question

How will you manage her?

Answer

- Patient has apparent temporal hollowing (Box A)
- Management involves: tailored history, examination, imaging and treatment options

3.2 Question

What are the potential causes of temporal hollowing?

Answer

- Trauma
- Iatrogenic: surgery (coronal flap), radiotherapy, botulinum toxin, temporalis hypertrophy or spasm
- Nutrition: generalised weight loss
- Autoimmune: connective tissue disease including Parry–Romberg
- Apparent: outward bowing of the zygomatic arch

3.3 Question

What are the key points in the history?

Answer

- Presenting complaint: temporal hollowing, bilateral, hair loss in area, progression
- Previous treatment: coronal flap to access zygomatic complex, previous treatment of hollowing, use of Botox
- Past medical history: previous irradiation, generalised weight loss, connective tissue disorder
- Assessment for surgery: anticoagulants, smoking, allergies, BMI as require fat if aiming for Coleman transfer

3.4 Question

What are the key points in the examination?

Answer

- Unilateral or bilateral temporal hollowing
- Incisions: e.g. coronal flap
- Scars
- Skin quality
- Does it reflect generalised low body weight?
- Zygomatic arch: is it more prominent due to previous fracture?
- Facial nerve (frontal branch) function
- Any suggestion of Parry–Romberg syndrome?

3.5 Question

What further information would you require to ascertain a diagnosis?

Answer

- Copies of any recent imaging, or request new CT scan
- Assess volume of soft tissues in temporal region
- Consider MRI scan

3.6 Question

The patient had a bicoronal flap and now has bitemporal hollowing. What are the treatment options?

Answer

- Do nothing and camouflage with hair style
- Patient-specific implant: reuse coronal flap but the implant is placed beneath the temporalis muscle and screwed into place and muscle resuspended
- Injectable fillers (Box B)
- Coleman fat transfer procedure

3.7 Question

The patient wants to go for autologous fillers. How would you advise the patient for this procedure?

Answer

- Fat is harvested from the abdomen or thigh (Box C)
- Potential complications can occur to both the donor and recipient sites (Box D)
- Poor outcomes in smokers
- Resorption rate <70%
- Procedure can be repeated if required

Box A: Pathophysiology of temporal hollowing

- A deficiency in the temporalis muscle or overlying temporal fat pad
- Due to ischaemia or denervation of the muscle or fat pad
- May result in loss of support to the eyebrow, leading to brow ptosis

---

Box B: Types of augmentation for temporal hollowing

- Injectable filler: autologous fat, bovine collagen, hyaluronic acid
- Implant: silicone, titanium mesh, polyetheretherketone (PEEK), methyl methacrylate

---

Box C: Brief methodology of autologous fat transfer

- Tumescent solution is infiltrated into donor site to aid liposuction and reduce haemorrhage
- Commonly utilised solutions include crystalloid with added epinephrine, hyalase, and local anaesthetic
- A stab incision is made and a cannula with syringe introduced
- Fat is aspirated using long sweeping motions
- Harvested fat is generally centrifuged and serum removed
- Following a stab incision, fat is injected subcutaneously in fan-shape from several directions with a special cannula
- Multiple passes of the cannula creating tubules of fat within the deficient site. Always over build to allow for resorption

---

Box D: Potential complications of autologous fat transfer

Donor site:
- Bowel perforation (abdomen)
- Numbness (leg)
- Haematoma

Recipient site:
- Lumpiness
- Overcorrection
- Facial nerve weakness

Further reading

Kim S, Matic DB. The anatomy of temporal hollowing: the superficial temporal fat pad. J Craniofac Surg 2005; 16:760–763.

Short case 4: LeFort III advancement

This patient returns to clinic three weeks post surgery to check on his progress.

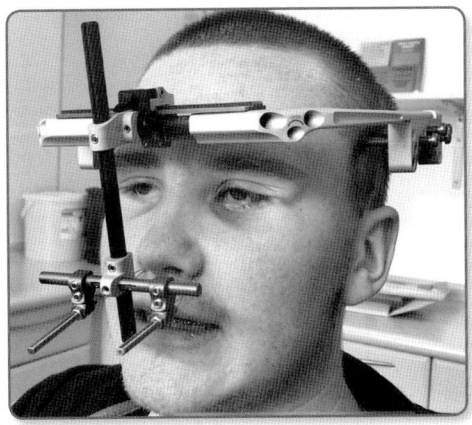

4.1 **Question**
Describe what you can see in this figure.

Answer
- Patient is in their 20s with external midface distractor in situ
- Frame used to perform midface distraction
- Coronal flap incision with cuts most probably at LeFort III level
- Good prominence of zygomas and step at ZF suture
- Possibly towards the end of the distraction phase

4.2 **Question**
How would you assess this patient?

Answer
- History
- Examination
- Plain films
- CT
- MRI: assess for raised ICP or Chiari malformation
- Study models
- Photographs

4.3 **Question**
What are the pertinent points in the history?

Answer
Preoperative:
- Airway: retruded midface, choanal atresia, sleeve trachea
- Corneal irritation

- Chewing
- Aesthetics: midface retrusion, malar flattening

Postoperative:
- Time since surgery
- number of turns per day
- Changes to facial appearance
- Airway
- Eyes
- Occlusion
- Gape: trismus from coronal flap and the cranial fixation pins through temporalis muscle
- VPI

4.4 Question

What are the pertinent points in the examination?

Answer

- Vector of advancement
- Tightness of wires and cranial fixation pins
- Healing of incisions: scalp, intraoral, lower eyelid (if used)
- Ophthalmic assessment
- Occlusion, airway, speech, nasal regurgitation (VPI)

4.5 Question

How does an external distractor frame work?

Answer

- Multivector: screws, nuts and bolts alter the vectors as midface is advanced
- Pins go into the scalp until finger tight
- Frame must remain symmetrical, with transverse bar above level of eyes and just away from skin
- Plates are attached to anterior maxilla
- Wires are passed transcutaneously and exit in perialar area
- Alternative fixation is to teeth or anterior maxilla with zygomatic and maxillary footplates, screws and rods
- The swivel clamps and spindles on horizontal carbon bar are turned until the wire is tight

4.6 Question

Where are the bone cuts made for a LeFort III distraction and how are they accessed?

Answer

- Coronal flap: access nasal bridge, frontozygomatic suture, orbital floor, medial and lateral orbital rim
- Lower eyelid approaches to orbital floors are described but not used in practice

4.7 Question

What are the components of distraction?

Answer

- Latent period: usually 3–4 days in adults
- Distraction: a single turn of 0.5 mm is performed twice a day. Generally, tend to over-correct
- Consolidation: for 8–12 weeks

4.8 Question

How does a monobloc advancement differ from a LeFort III osteotomy differ in technique and risks?

Answer

- Technique: moves the forehead/frontal bone, supraorbital bar and LeFort III segments as one unit (Box A and B)
- Risks: higher infection rates and greater blood loss than a LeFort III, due to communication between the cranial and nasal cavities (Box C)

Box A: Uses of LeFort III osteotomy

- Broadly used on two types of patient
- Nonsyndromic: genetic, postradiotherapy
- Syndromic: commonly Crouzon, Pfeiffer and Apert

Box B: Advantages of distraction over one-step osteotomy

- Larger advancement with greater control
- Shorter hospital stay
- Less complications
- Greater stability without the need for bone grafts
- Less relapse
- Better improvement in obstructive sleep apnoea
- Easier to assess VPI

Box C: Disadvantages of distraction over one-step osteotomy

- Compliance
- Damage to device may alter distraction vector
- Need a further operation under GA to remove plates and wires
- Overall treatment takes longer
- Cost of the distractor: single use in many countries

Further reading

Holmes AD, Wright GW, Meara JG, et al. LeFort III internal distraction in syndromic craniosynostosis. J Craniofac Surg 2002; 13:262–272.

Kaban LB, West B, Conover M, et al. Midface position after LeFort III advancement. Plast Reconstr Surg 1984; 73:758–767.

Short case 5: Zygomaticus implants

This patient who is well known to the department returns to clinic for routine follow-up.

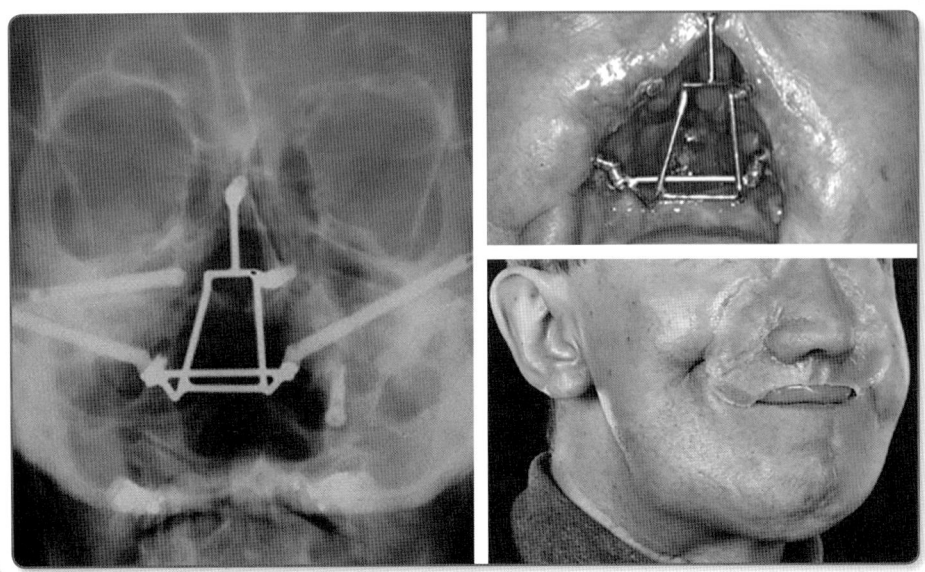

5.1 **Question**

How would you assess the patient in this figure, mindful of the PA radiograph?

Answer

- Patient has had zygomatic implant placement (Box A)
- Assessment comprises: tailored history, examination and, if indicated, imaging

5.2 **Question**

What are the key points in the follow-up history?

Answer

- Nasal discharge and pain over cheek: suggestive of sinusitis
- Alteration in cheek sensation: suggestive of infraorbital nerve damage
- Restriction or pain in ocular movements: suggestive of implant placement into the orbit
- Identify original indications for placement (Box B)

5.3 **Question**

What are the key points in the follow-up examination?

Answer

- Assess stability of prosthesis in situ

- Remove prosthesis if possible to assess potential bone loss, peri-implantitis and recurrence if an oncology case
- Eye assessment: if concerns about implant position

5.4 Question

What follow-up imaging would you perform and why?

Answer

- OPG: often taken postoperatively as a baseline to ascertain bone loss around implant
- CT: required to definitively ensure correct implant placement. Conventional CT instead of a CBCT enables assessment of potential sinusitis
- CBCT: can image up to and including the frontal sinus

5.5 Question

How are zygomatic implants placed?

Answer

- Most commonly performed under general anaesthesia or sedation
- Buccal sulcus horseshoe incision to deglove maxilla
- Lateral window is cut into maxillary sinus, preserving integrity of sinus lining
- Surgical guide or intra operative navigation may be used, but they are bulky
- Implant drills angled from the ridge aiming laterally upwards into zygomatic buttress
- Good evidence to suggest they can be immediately loaded

5.6 Question

What other options are there to zygomaticus implants?

Answer

- Sinus lift: for relatively small defects
- Bone graft: intraoral (volume may be insufficient) extraoral (potential additional morbidity)
- Short implants
- Implants into the pterygoid plates

Box A: Zygomaticus implants

- Long implant (generally 30–55 mm length)
- Anchors into the zygoma by passing through the maxillary sinus
- Generally used to retain a complete upper denture and/or facial prosthesis
- Can use straight or angled abutments (up to 60°)
- Typically, two to four zygomatic implants are used with or without two to four regular dental implants placed in the anterior maxilla
- Generally restored with either a fixed bridge or bar retained denture
- Published 95% survival rate after 10 years (Box C)

> **Box B: Indications for zygomaticus implants**
> - Severely resorbed edentulous maxilla
> - Failed sinus augmentation or bone graft
> - Rehabilitation after tumor resection or trauma composite defects of the maxilla and face
> - Failure after conventional implants

Further reading

Aparicio C, Manresa C, Francisco K, et al. The long-term use of zygomatic implants: a 10-year clinical and radiographic report. Clin Implant Dent Relat Res 2014; 16:447–459.

Glauser R, et al. Stability measurements of immediately loaded machined and oxidized implants in the posterior maxilla. A comparative clinical study using resonance frequency analysis. App Osseoint Res 2001; 4:1–5.

Long case 6: Arteriovenous vascular malformation

This patient complains of a long-term lump on his forehead that has recently increased in size following trauma (Box A).

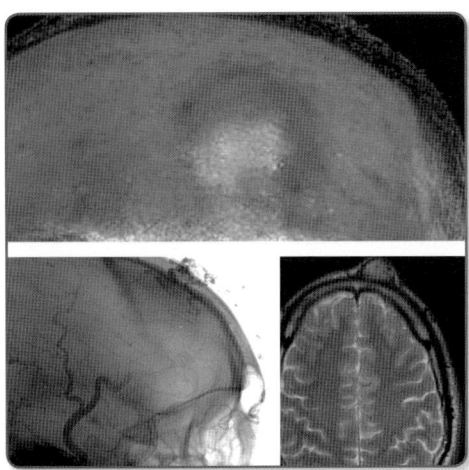

6.1 **Question**

How would you assess the patient shown in the figure?

Answer

Full assessment would comprise the following steps:
- Introduction and consent to assess (Box A)
- Patient positioning while cleaning hands and mentally come up with a spot diagnosis
- Tailored history
- Examination
- Review of any available investigations
- Summary back to the patient
- Differential diagnosis

6.2 **Question**

Why is it important to achieve an early diagnosis?

Answer

- A number of reasons for this presentation exist and include trauma, craniofacial and neoplastic (Box B)
- Care must be taken to ensure both history and examination covers all of these potential diagnoses and not to focus on one area

6.3 Question
What are the key points in the history?

Answer
- Presenting complaint: size increase, headaches, seizures
- History of complaint: present since a baby, trauma to frontal sinus, previous treatment and investigations
- Past medical and drug history
- Social history: cosmesis, affect on relationships

6.4 Question
How would you examine the patient?

Answer
- Inspection: size, colour
- Palpation: warmth, consistency, pulsatility, attachment to underlying tissues, underlying fractures
- Auscultation
- Transillumination
- Cranial nerve examination

6.5 Question
The lesion feels warm and pulsatile. What is the likely diagnosis?

Answer
- Most likely a vascular malformation (Box C)
- Of these, it is most likely a high flow arteriovenous malformation

6.6 Question
What first investigation would you request and why?

Answer
- Doppler ultrasound
- Confirm diagnosis as will demonstrate high flow
- Shows lesion consistency

6.7 Question
What would be your next examination?

Answer
- CT and MR angiogram are both valid options as they can both demonstrate size and potential intra cranial or intra orbital extension
- MR is nonionising (best seen in T2-weighted images, where blood appears white)
- CT demonstrates underlying fractures better

6.8 Question

Investigations confirm an AVM without intracranial extension. How would you manage the patient further?

Answer

- Staging of AVMs helps guide treatment (Box D). This case is most likely a Schobinger Stage II
- This lesion is best treated by embolisation followed by surgery (Box E)

Box A: Concept of a craniofacial long case

- A 15-minute assessment likely encompassing the structure above
- Patients with vascular malformations are easy to bring to the clinical examination
- Identifying the subtype of vascular malformation early will guide your management

---

Box B: Differential diagnosis of an isolated forehead lump

- Skin: epidermal cyst, dermoid cyst
- Fat: lipoma
- Blood: vascular malformation, organised haematoma.
- Bone: displaced frontal bone fracture, osteoma
- Other: frontal sinus mucocele

Box C: International Society for the Study of Vascular Anomalies (ISSVA) 2014 (Melbourne) classification

- Vascular tumours: benign (e.g. infantile haemangioma), locally aggressive (e.g. Kaposi sarcoma), malignant (e.g. angiosarcoma)
- Vascular malformations: simple (e.g. capillary), combined (e.g. lymphatico-venous)

Box D: Clinical Staging of AVMs (Schobinger 1990)

- I: Quiescent – arterial blush, warm
- II: Expansion – bruit, pulsatile
- III: Destruction – pain, ulceration, bleeding, infection
- IV: Decompensated

> **Box E: Management options for AVMs**
> - Conservative: threshold for treatment is Shobinger type III, but type II cases sometimes treated surgically
> - Embolisation alone: unusually done alone. Designed to obliterate nidus. Substances used include onyx, PHIL and Squid. Alcohol is rarely used and coils are only suitable for small AVMs
> - Embolisation plus surgery: surgery performed days to weeks later with an aim to completely excise the lesion
> - Surgery alone: for small lesions, or those affecting single aesthetic subunit, or palliative in extreme cases

Further reading

Mulliken JB, Glowacki J. Hemangiomas and vascular malformations in infants and children: a classification based on endothelial characteristics. Plast Reconstr Surg 1982; 69: 412–422.

Marler JJ, Mulliken JB. Vascular anomalies: classification, diagnosis, and natural history. Facial Plast Surg Clin North Am 2001; 9:495–504.

Mulligan PR, Prajapati HJ, Martin LG, Patel TH. Vascular anomalies: classification, imaging characteristics and implications for interventional radiology treatment approaches. Br J Radiol 2014; 87:20130392.

Chapter 10

Cleft lip and palate surgery

SHORT CASES

1. Cleft LeFort I osteotomy
2. Secondary cleft lip repair
3. Secondary cleft rhinoplasty

LONG CASE

4. Cleft palatal fistula with VPI

Short case 1: Cleft LeFort I osteotomy

This patient with a treated cleft lip returns to clinic for assesment of a potential osteotomy.

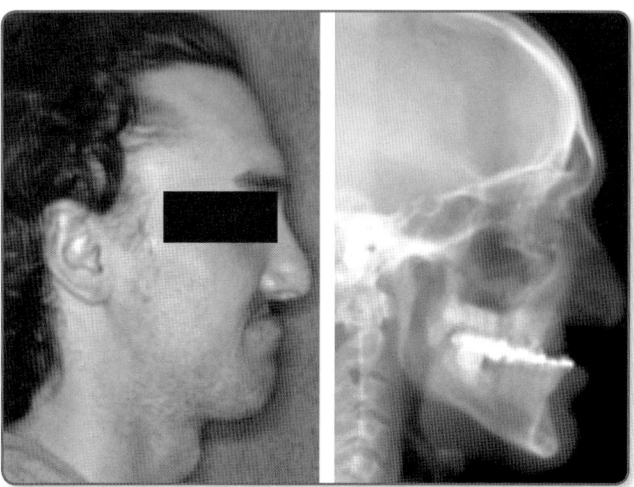

1.1 Question

What are the key features you would expect in your examination of the patient in the figure?

Answer

Extraoral:
- Facial asymmetry
- Nose: classical cleft features
- Lip: unilateral or bilateral cleft, repair type, maybe short
- Lack of or excessive upper incisor tooth show at rest and on smiling
- Tooth show asymmetry in unilateral cases with greater show on cleft side
- FMP angle: usually low
- Lower anterior facial height: usually low (maxillary vertical hypoplasia)
- Skeletal relationship: Class III (maxillary AP hypoplasia)
- Maxillary cant: rotation towards the lesser segment

Intraoral:
- Narrow palate (maxillary transverse hypoplasia)
- Orthodontic brackets
- Cleft of hard and/or soft palate
- Evidence of previous alveolar bone graft
- Missing or malformed teeth
- Presence of fistula
- Presurgical considerations: alignment, levelling and coordination of the arches, midline position correct surgically or orthodontically, decompensation

1.2 Question

How does the appearance of the incisors suggest what surgery the patient is likely to be having?

Answer

Incisors are decompensated and there is negative overjet:
- This suggests they will be having surgery and not orthodontic camouflage
- Patient is most likely planned for a LeFort 1 advancement and/or down grafting (Box A)

1.3 Question

What is the other option for advancing the maxilla?

Answer

- Distraction is alternative to traditional LeFort I advancement – can be either extraoral or intraoral (Box B and C)
- Rates of relapse and effects upon speech are comparable between distraction and LeFort I
- Only one small randomised controlled trial concerning the effectiveness of distraction osteogenesis compared to conventional orthognathic surgery exists

1.4 Question

What potential complications would you advise the patient to expect?

Answer

- Intraoperative: bleeding; unfavourable split if doing a BSSO as part of a bimaxillary procedure
- Early: infection and concurrent loss of bone graft (if grafted at the time); devitalisation of segment or teeth, malocclusion; worsening of hearing necessitating grommet insertion, widening of nose, rhinorrhea; oro-nasal fistula; numbness of cheeks, lips and gingiva (usually temporary); lower lip and tongue numbness if doing a BSSO as part of a bimaxillary procedure
- Late: nonunion or malunion of segments, relapse, worsened speech; permanent lip numbness

1.5 Question

What preoperative assessment is required?

Answer

- Psychological assessment to understand the patient's motivation for surgery
- Patient's expectations
- Perceptual speech assessment in combination with lateral videofluoroscopy to assess risk of developing VPI post-surgery
- Presence of existing pharyngeal flap does not increase risk of complications

1.6 Question

What is the role of the alveolar bone graft?

Answer

- Enable the canines/lateral incisors to erupt through viable bone ensuring the formation of a secure periodontal attachment around the tooth
- Enable orthodontic alignment of teeth
- Fuse the maxilla into a single segment to optimise orthodontic treatment and maxillary osteotomy if indicated
- Allow prosthetic replacement such as implants in those cases where lateral incisor is missing
- Close an oronasal fistula
- Create support for nose, alar base and lip

1.7 Question

What are the options if the alveolar bone graft has failed to fully unite the segments?

Answer

- Repeat secondary alveolar bone graft
- Segmental maxillary osteotomy to close gap

1.8 Question

When and how would you treat the nose?

Answer

- Secondary cleft septorhinoplasty is generally performed 6–12 months after orthognathic surgery
- At the time of orthognathic surgery inferior turbinates are often removed
- Little evidence to support a cinch suture

Box A: Aims of the cleft osteotomy

- Reduce alar hollowing
- Improve skeletal class III relationship
- Improve tip projection and nasal base support
- Change occlusion from class III to class I
- Improve incisor lip relationship
- Address occlusal cant

Box B: LeFort I surgery versus distraction

Advantages of LeFort I
- More cost-effective
- Single procedure
- No burden of distractors

Disadvantages of LeFort I
- Large movements are often required, which are more challenging to execute by doing a LeFort I
- Extensive scarring from previous surgery makes mobilisation difficult
- Abnormal anatomy with potential to comprise blood supply to premaxilla
- This is most challenging in bilateral cleft cases

Box C: Potential modifications to the osteotomy technique
- Smaller vestibular incisions to improve blood supply
- Sharp dissection of nasal floor from premaxilla on cleft side to reduce chances of causing an oro-nasal fistula
- Extensive mobilisation
- Adjunctive bone grafting
- Removal of inferior turbinate to increase nasal airflow
- Rigid fixation: may reduce relapse
- V to Y lip closure if lip short and/or large advancement

Further reading

Cheung LK, Chua HD, Hägg MR, et al. Cleft maxillary distraction versus orthognathic surgery: clinical morbidities and surgical relapse. Plast Reconstr Surg 2006; 118:996–1008.

Pereira VJ, Sell D, Tuomainen J, et al. Effect of maxillary osteotomy on speech in cleft lip and palate: perceptual outcomes of velopharyngeal function. Int J Lang Commun Disord 2013; 48:640–650.

Short case 2: Secondary cleft lip repair

The patient shown in this figure would like to know if there is anything that can be done to improve the appearance of their lip.

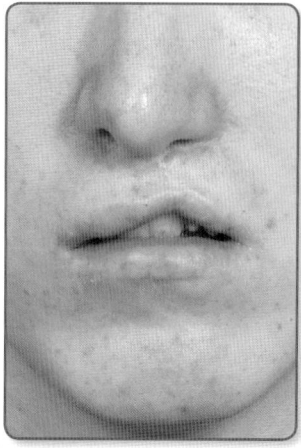

2.1 Question

How would you assess them?

Answer

- Lip scar is likely from a previous cleft repair
- Assessment comprises: history, examination and referral to psychology, performed in a multidisciplinary setting

2.2 Question

What information is relevant in the history?

Answer

- Age
- Reason for presentation: functional/aesthetic/both
- Clearly define which components of the lip appearance the patient does not like
- Previous revision surgery
- Presence of cleft palate
- Difficulty eating or speaking
- Planned orthognathic surgery
- Medical history including associated syndromes (e.g. van der Woude)
- Social history including school

Short case 2 Secondary cleft lip repair

2.3 Question
What are the key points in the examination?

Answer
- Lip repair type: often Millard, Fisher or Tennison in UK (Boxes B, C and D)
- Vermillion border: any stepping or irregularity
- Lip length: reduced or increased
- Lip mobility: discontinuity of obicularis oris
- Mucosa: excess or deficiency
- Scar: hypertrophic, irregular, pigmented
- Skeletal relationship
- Nose: alar base symmetry, columellar length

2.4 Question
At what age is primary cleft lip repair normally performed?

Answer
- Cleft lips are normally repaired within the first 6 months after birth
- If cleft extends into palate, this is repaired at same time (usually with a vomerine flap)
- Many hospital departments in the UK follow the Oslo protocol (Box A)

2.5 Question
What age would you ideally undertake any secondary lip surgery?

Answer
- No set age and timing for surgery
- Timing is determined by degree of psychological distress and deformity (Box E)
- Decision is determined in consultation with cleft clinical psychologist
- If performed before growth is complete then risk of needing further surgery, e.g. lip growth is usually complete by 14 years old
- If orthognathic surgery is planned then lip surgery should wait until completed as orthognathic surgery will probably affect lip position

2.6 Question
What type of surgery could help this patient?

Answer
- Patient requires full lip revision due to: lip shortness on the cleft side; lack of vermillion and wet/dry mucosa; whistle deformity caused by inadequate muscle reconstruction

Box A: Broad timings for primary unilateral cleft lip +/- palate repair based on the Oslo consensus

- Prenatal: potential diagnosis by ultrasound
- Birth: diagnosis. First contact. Attend "new baby MDT"
- 3–6 months: lip repair (Modified Millard (rotation – advancement), Fisher or Tennison) and vomerine flap to repair the hard palate in complete clefts of the lip and palate; in bilateral clefts of the lip and palate only one side of the hard palate will be closed at the first operation. This will then be followed by a second hard palate operation where a contralateral vomerine flap will be used to repair the hard palate cleft on the side left unrepaired at the first operation

Note: bilateral clefts need more operations to close the hard palate without compromising the blood supply to the premaxilla.

- 6–9 months: soft palate repair (Sommerlad technique)
- 18 months: 1st speech assessment
- 2 years: follow-up speech assessment if concerns at 18 months
- 3 years: multidisciplinary clinic appointment and 2nd speech assessment (for speech and language development and to assess velopharyngeal competence)
- Before 5 years: secondary speech surgery if velopharyngeal insufficiency diagnosed (before start school) to normalise speech before commencement of school-nature of surgery determined by findings on perceptual speech assessment and lateral videofluoroscopy (and less commonly nasoendoscopy)
- 8 years: 'secondary' alveolar bone graft-timing determined by root formation (1/2–2/3rds formed) of tooth being grafted for; may need pre-alveolar bone graft orthodontic treatment to expand collapsed arches and to create space to graft into
- 12 years: definitive orthodontic treatment once in the permanent dentition phase; definitive orthodontics delayed if orthognathic surgery a possibility
- 16 years: Commence orthodontics as part of orthognathic treatment plan
- 17–19 years: orthognathic surgery (LeFort I, bimax, segmental)
- 17 years onwards: revision of lip and/or septorhinoplasty (post-osteotomy)

Box B: Millard primary cleft lip repair

Advantages
- Scar mimics philtral column on cleft side
- Nasal sill is reconstructed
- "Cut as you go" philosophy meaning that modifications can be made during the procedure

Disadvantages
- May result in a short lip
- Scar crosses philtral column at nasal base

Box C: Tennison–Randall primary cleft lip repair

Advantages:
- Maintains lip length

Disadvantages:
- Scar crosses philtral column

Box D: Fisher primary lip repair

Advantages:
- Respects anatomical subunits
- Scar mimics philtrum

Disadvantages:
- Marking time consuming and intricate
- Difficult to determine position of alar base

Box E: Bilateral primary cleft lip repair

- No uniformity between units on the technique and timings for repair as well as nature of presurgical orthopaedics
- Some units repair both sides simultaneously, some will carry out a lip adhesion initially and some repair the lip on one side and then repair the other side later
- If repair is staged, the more severe side is repaired first, and the second side is repaired approximately 3–6 months later
- If repair both sides then often done with bilateral Millard flap

Further reading

Bhuskute A, Tollefson T. Cleft Lip Repair, Nasoalveolar Molding, and Primary Cleft Rhinoplasty. Facial Plast Surg Clin North Am 2016; 24:453–466.

Fisher DM. Unilateral cleft lip repair: An anatomical subunit approximation technique. Plast Reconstr Surg 2005; 116:61–71.

Millard DR. Extensions of the rotation-advancement principle for wide unilateral cleft lips. Plast Reconstr Surg 1968; 42:535–544.

Monson L, Khechoyan DY, Buchanan EP, Hollier LH Jr, et al. Secondary lip and palate surgery. Clin Plast Surg 2014; 41:301–309.

Mulliken JB. Primary repair of bilateral complete cleft lip and nasal deformity. Plast Reconstr Surg 2001; 108:181–194.

Sommerlad BC. A technique for cleft palate repair. Plast Reconstr Surg 2003; 112:1542–1548.

Zhang JX, Arneja JS. Evidence-Based Medicine: The Bilateral Cleft Lip Repair. Plast Reconstr Surg 2017; 140:152e–165e.

Short case 3: Secondary cleft rhinoplasty

The patient shown in the figure attends clinic asking for surgery on their nose.

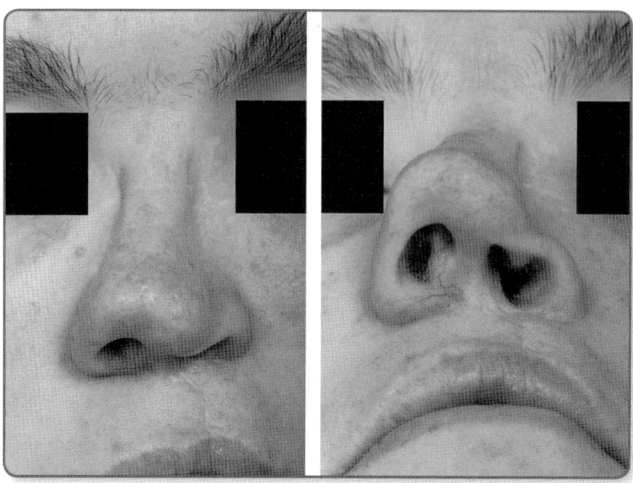

3.1 Question

How would you assess them?

Answer

- Assessment involves history, examination, assessment of airway patency and nasendoscopy – performed in a multidisciplinary setting with cleft psychology input

3.2 Question

What are key points in the history?

Answer

- Reason for attendance: psychosocial, aesthetic, functional, complications
- Aesthetic: overall appearance, nostril asymmetry, tip projection, alar asymmetry, alar base discrepancies, septal deviation
- Functional: difficulty breathing, especially during exercise
- Complications: chronic rhinosinusitis
- Sleep: airway blockage due to septal deviation so may lie on side of least patent airway
- Previous secondary surgery (Box C)
- Planned orthognathic surgery
- General medical health
- Social history: progress at school, future plans

3.3 Question
What are the key examination features in the cleft nose?

Answer
- Front: nasal bone position, nasal width, alar position and symmetry, tip appearance and projection (Boxes A and B)
- Side: nasal height in relation to facial thirds, nasal projection, columella show, alar position, nasolabial angle, shape of nasal dorsum
- Above: dorsum and tip position
- Below: alar base, position, columella height and symmetry, septal deviation, alar shape
- Intranasal: septal deviation, turbinate condition

3.4 Question
How is airway potency assessed in clinic?

Answer
- Cottle's manoevre can be used to assess the internal nasal valve
- Stand behind patient
- Get patient to breath in and out and listen
- Occlude one nostril by pressing on ala only
- Breath in and out and look for indentation in ala
- Pull cheek away on other side of where occluding nostril and this opens the airway more

3.5 Question
When is rhinoplasty generally performed?

Answer
- Primary rhinoplasty is generally at same time as the lip (within 6 months)
- Early secondary is generally performed prior to starting school (Box D)
- Secondary rhinoplasty should be performed after completion of skeletal nasal growth (>17 years old)
- If maxillary osteotomy is planned it should be delayed until after this

3.6 Question
What are the likely principles of secondary nasal repair in this patient?

Answer
- Open tip approach to increase access
- Alar base repositioning: often using a V to Y plasty
- Centralisation of the cartilaginous septum
- Osteotomy of vomer and nasal bones

- Repositioning of lower alar cartilage after skeletonisation of cartilage by dissecting cartilage free from both skin and nasal mucosa
- Nasal valve reconstruction
- Columellar strut to increase tip projection

Box A: Clinical features of the nose in unilateral clefts

- Often have thickened sebaceous skin
- Tip asymmetry
- Ala base: lies inferior or superior, posterior and lateral on the cleft side
- Anterior nasal spine: deviated away from cleft side
- Dorsum deviated away from cleft side
- Septum deviated away from the cleft side caudally
- Columella shortened on the cleft side
- Collapse of the alar cartilage on the cleft side
- Missing or hypoplastic nasal sill
- Nasolabial angle: decreased
- Tip: flattened, bifid, widened
- Maxillary hypoplasia: on cleft side
- Turbinates: inevitably hypertrophic on noncleft side

Box B: Clinical features of the nose in bilateral clefts

- Bilateral widening of the alar bases
- Vomer, septum and dorsum remains in the midline
- Columella shortened
- Widened often bifid tip
- Bilateral maxillary hypoplasia

Box C: Primary cleft rhinoplasty

- Carried out at same time as primary lip repair
- The technique used varies widely among cleft surgeons
- One of the most common approaches was originally described by McComb and later modified by Salyer
- Uses the same incisions as those to access the lip
- The ala is released from the piriform
- The skin is elevated from the surface of the middle and lateral alar cartilages
- The lower lateral cartilage is suspended superomedially by a transcutaneous suture

---

Box D: Early secondary cleft rhinoplasty

- The aim of primary repair is to not require further treatment
- However, approximately 10% of patients require revision rhinoplasty
- Early secondary cleft rhinoplasty is generally performed prior to starting school to increase confidence and is only performed rarely
- Access may be via a rim incision in milder cases but usually through a trans-columella open tip approach

Further reading

Allori A, Mulliken J. Evidence-Based Medicine: Secondary Correction of Cleft Lip Nasal Deformity. Plast Reconstr Surg 2017; 140:166e–176e.

Marcus J, Allori A, Santiago P. Principles of Cleft Lip Repair: Conventions, Commonalities, and Controversies. Plast Reconstr Surg 2017; 139:764e–780e.

Salyer K, Xu H, Genecov E. Unilateral cleft lip and nose repair; closed approach Dallas protocol completed patients. J Craniofac Surg 2009; 20:1939–1955.

Long case 4: Cleft palatal fistula with VPI

The patient shown in this figure is complaining of problems with their speech.

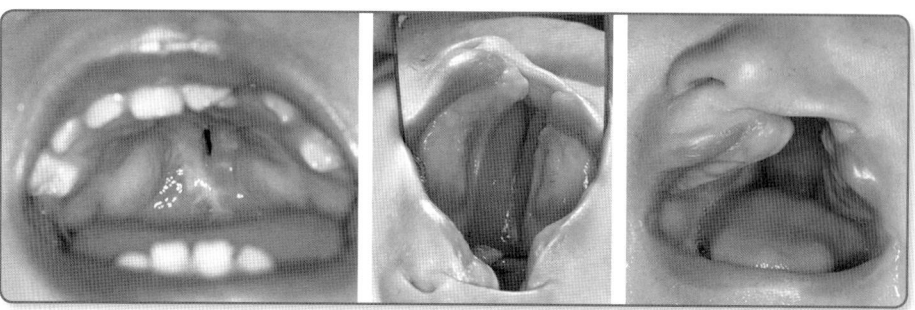

4.1 Question
What are the key points in the history?

Answer
- Previous repairs: age (Box A), type (Box B), complications
- Speech: perceptual speech assessment
- Nasal regurgitation
- Ears: hearing, infections
- General medical health
- Social history: school

4.2 Question
What are the key points in the examination?

Answer
- Lip: repair type
- Palate: repair type
- Fistula location: anterior, midpalatal, soft/hard palate junction, hard palate
- Fistula size: small (<2 mm), medium (3–5 mm) or large (>5 mm)
- Perceptual speech assessment: hypernasality, nasal airflow errors, cleft speech characteristics
- Nasometry

4.3 Question
On examination the patient has a small hard palate fistula; on perceptual speech assessment the patient has hypernasality and nasal turbulence; nasometry reveals increased nasalance score. What is the patient's diagnosis and how would you assess them further?

Answer
- The patient has velopharyngeal insufficiency (VPI)

- Likely due to a combination of effects of palatal oro-nasal fistula (Box C) and velopharyngeal incompetence
- Further investigations needed are lateral videofluoroscopy and a review of results with surgeon and speech therapist in MDT clinic

4.4 Question

What is VPI and what may cause it?

Answer

- VPI occurs when the soft palate does not make contact with the posterior pharyngeal wall during speech (Box C)
- Nasal air escape during speech gives rise to hypernasality (speech produced with excessive resonance within the nasal cavity)
- Nasal emission can also be caused by an oro-nasal fistula

4.5 Question

How would you treat this patient?

Answer

- Surgery is recommended for VPI and it should be performed more than 6 months after any previous surgery (Box B)
- The figure shows a hard palatal defect that is not too large to close primarily (Box D)
- Two-layer tension free closure is most successful
- In those cases where not possible to close the fistula using local flaps then local pedicled flaps in form of buccinator myomucosal flaps or tongue flaps are most common options

4.6 Question

What are the potential complications of palatal fistula repair?

Answer

- Flap necrosis
- Fistula recurrence (relates to size but 20% recur)
- Worsened speech
- Worsened nasal fluid and food regurgitation

4.7 Question

If the cause of VPI had been felt to be the soft palate, what is required before?

Answer

- Functional assessment: to determine soft palate during speech and swallowing
- Videofluoroscopy and nasendoscopy: to determine soft palate length and extensibility, the size and position of the VP gap and the position of the levator veli palatini muscles within the soft palate

4.8 Question

If the palate is moving on phonation and the muscles are positioned posteriorly but the palate is short, what are the treatment options?

Answer
- Palatal lengthening in the form of an oral z-plasty, a Furlow procedure or bilateral buccinator flaps to lengthen the palate
- Hynes procedure to bring the posterior pharyngeal wall forward
- Other options include the sphincter pharyngoplasty (Orticochea of Jackson) or midline pharyngeal flap pharyngoplasty (Box E)

Box A: Palatal cleft surgery

- The aim of palate repair is to repair the cleft and in so doing close the cleft and create a functional velopharyngeal port so as to enable normal speech production, prevent fluid and food regurgitation into the nose while eating and to prevent middle ear infections
- Primary repair is undertaken before the age of 1 year
- Early secondary repair is undertaken prior to school going age, i.e. before the age of 5 years in the UK
- Incidence of palatal fistula formation is approximately 10–15%

Box B: Primary hard and soft palate repair options

- Hard palate: vomer flap (in complete CLP), Von Langenbeck repair, Bardach, Sommerlad
- Soft palate: Sommerlad radical muscle dissection, Furlow double opposing Z-plasty

---

Box C: Aetiology of velopharyngeal insufficiency

- Insufficient tissue: short palate (cleft patients), oro-nasal fistulae, post adenoidectomy, trauma
- Neurological: neurofibromatosis, cerebral palsy, stroke
- Mislearning: hearing impairment

Box D: Secondary hard palate (e.g. oro-nasal fistula) defect treatment options

Small defects – "inkwell" incision with turnover flaps (pedicled nasally) to close the nasal layer and then von Langenbeck incisions and medial advancement of the oral flaps bilaterally to close the oral layer; to prevent re-fistulisation the use of an interpositional graft between the newly constructed nasal and oral layer either in the form of autogenous ear cartilage (gold standard) or alloplastic material (PDS sheet) is recommended:
- Transposition flaps pedicled on the greater palatine vessels
- Buccal fat pad
- Tongue flap
- Buccinator flap: mucosa only or muscle plus mucosa
- Facial artery myomucosal flap (FAMM)
- Free flap (for large fistulae)
- Obturator where surgery is not possible or indicated

> **Box E: Secondary soft palate repair treatment options**
> - Palatal re-repair: if palate of adequate length but levator muscles situated anteriorly
> - Oral z-plasty: if palate short (small gap) and levator muscles situated posteriorly
> - Furlow double opposing z-plasty: for small gap
> - Buccinator flaps: if palate short (large gap) and levator muscles situated posteriorly
> - Hynes pharyngoplasty: if palate short and there is no history of obstructive breathing
> - Sphincter pharyngoplasty (Orticochea or Jackson): if palate functioning well but lateral nasopharyngeal gaps on nasoendoscopy
> - Midline pharyngeal flap: if nasopharyngeal gap is in midline on nasoendoscopy

Further reading

Hodgins N, Hoo C, McGee P, Hill C. A survey of assessment and management of velopharyngeal incompetence (VPI) in the UK and Ireland. J Plast Reconstr Aesthet Surg 2015; 68:485–491.

Chapter 11

Facial aesthetic surgery

SHORT CASES

1. Nonsurgical cosmetic treatment
2. Rhytidectomy (facelift)
3. Facial reanimation
4. Upper blepharoplasty
5. Post-traumatic scar management

LONG CASE

6. Dorsal nasal hump

Short case 1: Nonsurgical cosmetic treatment

This patient attends your private clinic wanting a cosmetic solution to her forehead wrinkles.

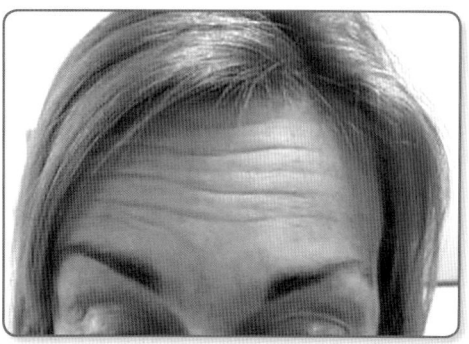

1.1 Question

What are the key features to be aware when examining the patient shown in this figure?

Answer

- Distinguish between static and dynamic wrinkles
- Static wrinkles are present at rest and respond best to fillers
- Dynamic wrinkles appear on movement and are best treated with botulinum toxin

1.2 Question

How does botulinum toxin work?

Answer

- Neurotoxin produced by Clostridium botulinum strains with multiple subtypes (Box A)
- Cleaves a protein responsible for the release of acetylcholine into the neuromuscular synapse
- Onset of action is delayed (peak effect 7–10 days) and temporary

1.3 Question

What are the possible complications of botulinum toxin?

Answer

- Haematoma, dissatisfaction
- Mask-like appearance from overestimation of dose and/or widespread injections

- Headache
- Ptosis and/or diplopia from wrong site injection near the orbital rim

1.4 Question
What are the different types of fillers?

Answer
- Most popular fillers are hyaluronic acid (HA) dermal fillers (e.g. Juvederm): products vary according to the ratio of high to low molecular weight HA particles (e.g. Voluma XC is thicker than Vollure XC)
- Greater longevity found using fillers based on bovine collagen (e.g. Zyderm), some with additives such as inert polymethylmethacrylate (PMMA) beads (e.g. Artecoll)
- Other constituents for microspheres include calcium hydroxyapatite (e.g. Radiesse)
- Constituents such as poly-L-lactic acid (e.g. Sculptra) may stimulate the body's own production of collagen, achieving longer lasting effects

1.5 Question
What are the possible complications of fillers?

Answer
- Haematoma
- Skin necrosis: injection too superficial or inadvertent intravascular injection
- Uneven result
- Dissatisfaction
- Hypersensitivity responses
- Chronic infection
- Hypertrophic scars
- Granulomas
- Blindness from embolisation of filler particles

1.6 Question
What are the roles of dermabrasion and microdermabrasion?

Answer
- Both are techniques to rejuvenate the skin
- Dermabrasion uses a rotary handpiece to remove skin up to as deep as the reticular dermis with profound effects
- Microdermabrasion in contrast uses inert crystals (e.g. aluminium oxide)
- It removes the stratum corneum and stimulates elastin and collagen formation, along with increased myofibroblast migration

Box A: Types of botulinum toxin

- There are eight different exotoxins but type A is available for cosmetic use
- Whilst there is a wide remit of applications (blepharospasm, torticollis, spasticity in cerebral palsy or stroke and masseteric hypertrophy to name but a few), its use in nonsurgical cosmetic treatment have traditionally been 'off-licence'
- Whilst Botox was licensed for cosmetic use in the US in 2002, it was licensed for treating glabellar lines as Vistabel in the UK in 2006
- Dysport is marketed for cosmetic use under the name Azzalure in the UK as of 2009
- Importantly, Speywood units between the major brands are not interchangeable and different brands also exhibit different patterns of spread

Box B: Chemical peels

- These remove upper layers of skin by inflicting a controlled clinical burn to a particular layer
- Stratum basale: superficial, e.g. Jessner's solution
- Epidermal-papillary level: medium, e.g. trichloroacetic acid 20–35%
- Reticular dermis: deep, e.g. trichloroacetic acid 45–50%

Box C: Skincare and Obagi

- Prescription-only skincare products often form part of a standard nonsurgical cosmetic practice
- Tretinoin or all-trans retinoic acid (ATRA) is a vitamin A derivative, which can increase epidermal thickness and stratum corneum compaction
- These are most notably combined with benzoyl peroxide, zinc oxide and 4% hydroquinone
- They prevent discoloration and treat hyperpigmentation in Obagi products such as Nu-Derm

Further reading

De Maio M, Swift A, Signorini M, et al. Facial assessment and injection guide for botulinum toxin and injectable hyaluronic acid fillers: focus on the upper face. Plast Reconstr Surg 2017; 140:265e–276e.

De Maio M, Wu WTL, Goodman GJ, et al. Facial assessment and injection guide for botulinum toxin and injectable hyaluronic acid fillers: focus on the lower face. Plast Reconstr Surg 2017; 140:393e–404e.

El-Domyati M, Hosam W, Abdel-Azim E, et al. Microdermabrasion: a clinical, histometric and histopathologic study. J Cosmet Dermatol 2016; 15:503–513.

Lazzeri D, Agostini T, Figus M, et al. Blindness following cosmetic injections of the face. Plast Reconstr Surg 2012; 129:995–1012.

Short case 2: Rhytidectomy (facelift)

This patient is requesting a facelift.

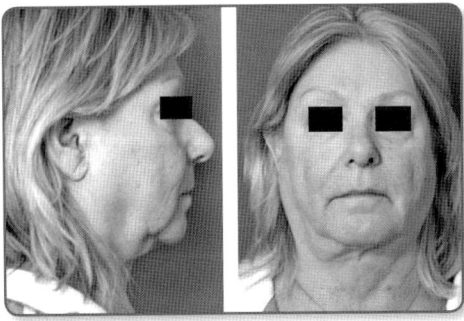

2.1 Question

What are the key features in the history of this patient?

Answer

- Establish exact concerns
- Smoking status and use of anticoagulants
- Previous facial surgery

2.2 Question

What are the key examination features?

Answer

- Skin quality: assess whether adjuvant measure to improve skin quality are required, e.g. Obagi, chemical peels or dermabrasion
- Hairline to plan incisions: pre or retrotragal; pretrichial or within hairline
- Assess whether patient requires adjuvant surgical procedures, e.g. blepharoplasty, platysmaplasty
- Loss of cervicomental angle for signs of aging (Box A)

2.3 Question

What is SMAS and how is it managed during a facelift?

Answer

- SMAS is the superficial musculoaponeurotic system (Box B)
- Classic facelift: SMAS is incised as inverted L and redraped posterosuperiorly
- SMAS-ectomy: removing a line of SMAS from lateral canthus to angle of mandible
- SMAS-plication: a dog-ear is taken anteriorly to provide malar fullness where desired

- Extended SMAS: takes the anterior dissection over the zygomaticus major – this releases deeper ligamentous attachments in midface allowing for vertical suspension of malar fat pad and aims to efface nasolabial fold
- Composite rhytidectomy: is a modification of the extended SMAS to include the suspension of the lower orbicularis oculi

2.4 Question

What is a MACS lift?

Answer

- Short scar approach is used
- Running sutures used in a vertical vector and anteroinferiorly to gather the SMAS and anchor it to deep temporal fascia
- Vector is predominantly vertical

2.5 Question

What is an S-lift?

Answer

- Involves pre-excision of skin (technically challenging), combined with purse-string sutures from SMAS to periosteum (Box C)

2.6 Question

What are possible complications of rhytidectomy?

Answer

- Haematoma
- Greater auricular nerve paresthesia/numbness
- Facial nerve weakness: persistent in up to 2–3% affecting marginal mandibular nerve most commonly
- Infection
- Wound dehiscence
- Scars
- Ear distortion and 'pixie' ear deformity due to careless in setting of skin flap

---

Box A: Key features of aging

- Forehead/glabellar rhytids
- Brow ptosis
- Dermatochalasis of the eyelids +/– lid laxity +/– lacrimal gland/fat herniation/festoons
- Nasojugal/palpebromalar/mid-cheek grooves and nasolabial fold deepening
- Perioral wrinkles
- Jowls
- Platysmal bands

> **Box B: Key terminology for facelifts in terms of SMAS**
> - SMAS is key to achieving a lasting 'pull' in the vector(s) of choice; continue with the temporoparietal fascia above and the platysma below
> - Composite flap: the concept of raising skin and SMAS together
> - MACS lift: a minimal access cranial suspension technique
> - Short scar facelift: the approach is restricted to the preauricular region, limiting the vector to a vertical pull

> **Box C: A history of facelifts**
> - 1912: Hollander describes first facelift
> - 1960: Aufricht described deeper suturing incorporating SMAS
> - 1974: Skoog describes deeper dissection
> - 1979: Tessier describes a subperiosteal release
> - 1989: Furnas identifies midfacial ligaments
> - 1990: Hamra describing the deep plane rhytidectomy with release of ligamentous attachments
> - 1999: Saylan describes minimally invasive S-lift
> - 2001: Short scar facelift described by Baker
> - 2002: MACS lift described by Tonnard

Further reading

Barrett DM, Gerecci D, Wang TD. Facelift controversies. Facial Plast Surg Clin N Am 2016; 24: 357–366.

Hamra ST. The deep-plane rhytidectomy. Plast Reconstr Surg 1990; 86:53–61.

Prado A, Andrades P, Danilla S, Castillo P, Leniz P. A clinical retrospective study comparing two short-scar face lifts: minimal access cranial suspension versus lateral SMASectomy. Plast Reconstr Surg 2006; 117:1413–1425.

Tonnard P, Verpaele A, Monstrey S, et al. Minimal access cranial suspension lift: a modified S-lift. Plast Reconstr Surg 2002; 109:2074–2086.

Short case 3: Facial reanimation

The patient shown in the figure returns to clinic.

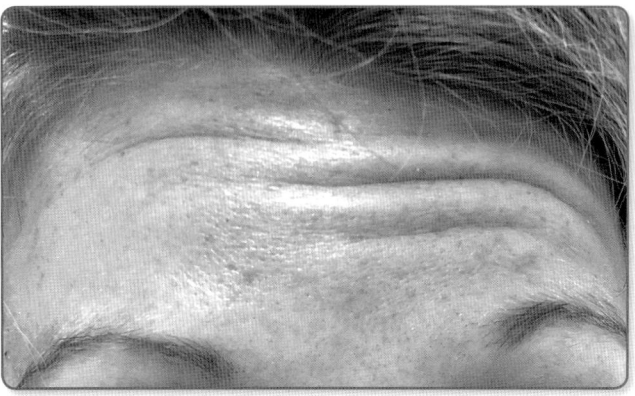

3.1 Question
What are the most common causes of facial palsy?

Answer
- Bell's palsy
- Benign/malignant tumours
- Iatrogenic injury
- Varicella-Zoster
- Traumatic injury
- Congenital palsy

3.2 Question
What are the key examination features?

Answer
- Facial asymmetry: this should be graded (Box A) and classified (Box B)
- Paralytic lagophthalmos and/or exposure keratopathy
- Eyelid retraction and/or ectropion
- Nasal valve collapse
- Oral incompetence
- Dysarthria

3.3 Question
What are static repairs, and give some examples?

Answer
- Treatment options broadly categorized as static or dynamic
- Static methods do not restore function but improve resting appearance

- Static techniques include: tensor fascial lata slings to the oral commissure, rhytidectomies, contralateral depressor labii inferioris/depressor anguli oris resection (or chemodenervation), tarsorrhaphy, eyelid weights and brow lifts

3.4 Question

What dynamic repair options are available and what determines which one you would choose?

Answer

- Dynamic repair options are determined by timing (Box C)
- The ideal is direct neurorrhaphy at the time of injury/resection with interpositional nerve grafts where warranted (e.g. greater auricular nerve, sural nerve, thoracodorsal nerve)
- Cross-facial nerve grafts (CFNG) may be used where denervation has been present for <18 months and viable musculature remains
- Where nonviable facial muscle is present, temporalis transfer may be utilised or free tissue transfer such as gracilis muscle
- Options for 'coaption' (drawing together) with the donor site nerve include either CFNG (with the aim of achieving spontaneity) or other recipient site nerves such as masseteric or hypoglossal nerves
- Two stage procedures using CFNG with maximal neural ingrowth prior to free tissue transfer is probably the most popular option currently

3.5 Question

What do you understand by the terms 'baby-sitting' and 'neural supercharging'?

Answer

- Baby-sitting: using hypoglossal fibres to maintain healthy mimetic muscles until a CFNG has been developed to provide innervation to paralysed side
- Supercharging: provides dual innervation to obtain quantity of stimulus (hypoglossal) and quality (CFNG) combined

---

Box A: Grading systems

- American Academy of Otolaryngology-Head and Neck Surgery (AAO-HNS) Grading System 1.0 (House-Brackmann)
- A 6-point grading scale originally designed for grading palsy following vestibular schwannoma resection
- It lacks zonal descriptors and demonstrating poor interobserver variability
- Sunnybrook scale: a continuous scale sensitive to fine differences, which also accounts for synkinesis
- AAO-HNS Facial Nerve Grading System 2.0: adapted House–Brackmann scale including regional scoring system and accountings for synkinesis

> **Box B: Classification**
> - Facial palsy may be broadly categorised as flaccid facial palsy (FFP) or nonflaccid facial palsy (NFFP) when characterised by zonal variation in hypo- and hyperactivity +/- synkinesis
> - FFP can further be defined as acute or persistent with viable or nonviable musculature

> **Box C: CFNG versus other sources of innervation**
> - Potential drawbacks of such grafts include the small stimulus, the possibility of creating a segmental paralysis in the healthy donor hemiface and the slow growth (estimated 1–2 mm/day)
> - It is rare for more than 2 CFNGs to be used
> - The hypoglossal nerve poses issues such as donor site morbidity (dysphagia/dysarthria) and the absence of an emotional, spontaneous smile
> - The masseteric nerve presents less donor site morbidity but again the need for physiotherapy to achieve a 'natural' response

Further reading

Biglioi F. Facial reanimations: part II – long-standing paralyses. Br J Oral Maxillofac Surg 2015; 53:907–912.

Biglioli F. Facial reanimations: part I – recent paralyses. Br J Oral Maxillofac Surg 2015; 53:901–906.

Fujiwara T, Matsuda K, Kubo T, et al. Axonal supercharging technique using reverse end-to-side neurorrhaphy in peripheral nerve repair: an experimental study in the rat model. Neurosurgery 2007; 107:821–829.

Jowett N, Hadlock TA. An evidence-based approach to facial reanimation. Facial Plast Surg Clin N Am 2015; 23:313–334.

Kim L, Byrne PJ. Controversies in contemporary facial reanimation. Facial Plast Surg Clin N Am 2016; 24:275–297.

Short case 4: Upper blepharoplasty

The patient in the figure attends your private consultation clinic asking if anything can be done about the appearance of her eyes.

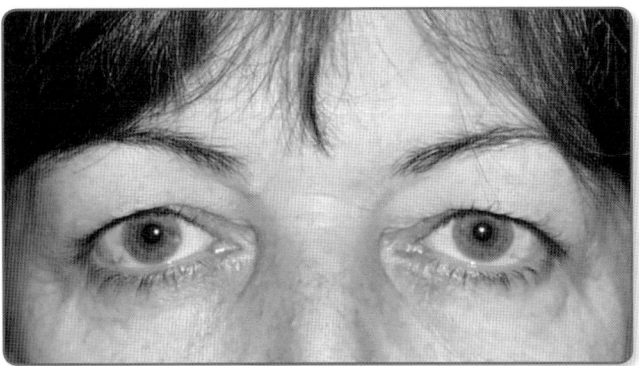

4.1 Question

What are the key features in the initial history taken from the patient presenting with the appearance shown in this figure?

Answer

- Specific concerns in terms of appearance
- Identify problems with vision: e.g. glaucoma, previous laser surgery, contact lens use, blepharitis, dry eyes
- Relevant medical history:
  - Diabetes
  - Connective tissue disease
  - Thyroid disease
  - Clotting disorders

4.2 Question

What are the key examination features?

Answer

- Examine for dermatochalasis (Box A)
- Any fat prolapse
- Any lateral fullness indicating lacrimal gland prolapse
- Coexisting ptosis (MRD1 <2 mm)
- 'Compensated brow ptosis' (Box B)

4.3 Question

You agree to perform blepharoplasty. What other procure may be required?

Answer

- Compensated brow ptosis may require a concomitant brow lift (Box C)

4.4 Question
How is the skin resection estimated?

Answer
- The 'pinch' test identifies the amount of lax skin that can be safely removed
- Lower limit of skin removal should be drawn 10–12 mm above the central eyelid margin and tapered to 5–6 mm above the lid margin medially and laterally
- Should be extended out towards the lateral brow from 3–8 mm beyond lateral commissure
- End result should be maintenance of a minimum of 20 mm skin between lash line and upper eyebrow

4.5 Question
How should the fat component be managed intraoperatively?

Answer
- Skin is removed with muscle leaving orbital septum exposed
- Gentle pressure on the globe will 'reveal' areas of fat herniation and septum is opened to deliver these
- Should not be excessive traction on the fat, as this risks overzealous removal, resulting in a 'skeletal' appearance
- Laterally, the lacrimal gland may need to be resuspended to periosteum if ptotic

4.6 Question
What are possible complications of blepharoplasty?

Answer
- Eyelid haematoma
- Retrobulbar haemorrhage
- Lagophthalmos
- Residual redundant skin
- Asymmetric or irregular eyelid creases
- Transient diplopia
- Strabismus if extraocular muscles damaged
- Corneal abrasion

Box A: Key terminology for eye assessment

- Dermatochalasis: excess laxity of skin
- MRD1: the margin reflex distance between the light reflex and central upper eyelid margin in millimeters
- MRD2: the distance from the light reflex to the central lower eyelid
- MLD: margin limbal distance, measuring from inferior point of limbus to central upper eyelid in extreme upgaze to quantify to ptosis

Box B: Compensated brow ptosis

- Facial cosmetic surgery should be assessed as a 'package' as patients rarely have isolated problems in a single area
- A classic example of this is compensated brow ptosis where ptosis is compensated for by the action of the frontalis
- In these patients, blepharoplasty alone can worsen their appearance
- This allows the eyes to remain open with relaxation of the frontalis muscle, thereby dropping the brow, which was previously raised to compensate!

Box C: Types of brow lift

- Direct: elliptical skin and muscle excision directly above the eyebrow; typically for male patients with thick eyebrows
- Mid-forehead: rarely used and dependent on deep rhytids in this region to conceal scar
- Pretrichial: just anterior to hairline
- Coronal: within hairline as per standard coronal flap
- Endoscopic: subperiosteal dissection endoscopically and 'up-cutting' to divide periosteum +/– corrugator/procerus; secured with monocortical screws or devices such as Endotine
- Transpalpebral: done via upper blepharoplasty approach

Further reading

Dutton JJ. Upper eyelid blepharoplasty with fat excision. In: Atlas of Oculoplastic and Orbital Surgery. Lippincott Williams & Wilkons, Philadelphia PA. 2013.

Yang P, Ko AC, Kikkawa DO, et al. Upper eyelid blepharoplasty: evaluation, treatment and complication minimization. Semin Plast Surg 2017; 31:51–57.

Short case 5: Post-traumatic scar management

This patient returns to clinic following a request from his general practitioner wondering if anything can be done to improve the appearance of his facial scarring.

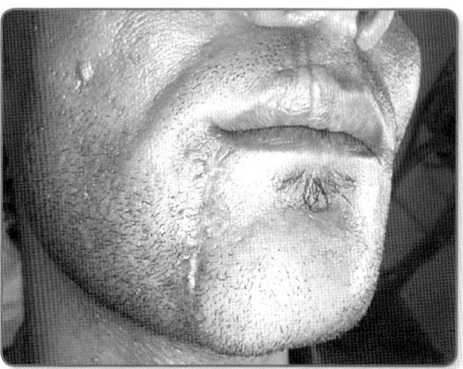

5.1 Question
What are the key features when examining the patient shown in this figure?

Answer
- Dimensions of the scar
- Any abnormalities, e.g. hypertrophic scar, keloid formation (Box A)
- The 'lie' of the scar and any scope for reorientation
- Contour discrepancy
- Colour mismatch/depigmentation

5.2 Question
What intraoperative techniques can be performed to reduce scar size?

Answer
- Incision-perpendicular to relaxed skin tension lines
- Atraumatic tissue handling
- Smallest diameter needle and suture size
- Tension-free closure
- Layered repair
- Wound edge eversion
- Good haemastasis

5.3 Question
What postoperative measures can be used to reduce scar size?

Answer
- Massage using an emollient: soften and mobilise the scar
- Silicone sheets: may help flatten scars but require compliance to wear for 23 h/day

5.4 Question
What nonsurgical options exist for managing keloid scars?

Answer

- Camoflague
- Intralesional injection of steroid (e.g. Kenalog, triamcinolone acetonide) to 'flatten' scar
- Intralesional excision to reduce possibility of recurrence
- Electron beam radiation therapy as an adjunct to surgical excision
- Mitomycin C, 5-fluorouracil and bleomycin
- Silicone sheeting and/or pressure garments

5.5 Question
When should scars be revised?

Answer

- No agreement in the literature exists
- Ample time should be allowed for spontaneous improvement
- Revision should be delayed if reasons for poor healing exist, e.g. nutritional deficiency, infection, high tension, smoking
- Collagen remodelling means scars take 12–18 months to mature and gain tensile strength of 70–80% of uninjured skin
- Revision of immature scars often cause hypertrophy and poor aesthetics

5.6 Question
In which scenarios would you consider early scar revision?

Answer

- Scars that can be improved by resurfacing
- Scars that have the potential to cause retraction of sensitive anatomical areas (e.g. lower eyelid)
- It remains unusual to revise any scar before 3 months

5.7 Question
What are the surgical options for scar revision?

Answer

- Straightforward excision
- Scar irregularisation
- Geometric broken lines closure
- Running W-plasty, Z-plasty: to reorient and/or lengthen
- Subcision: releasing tethered dermis

5.8 Question
What is autologous platelet-rich plasma and what is it used for?

Answer

- Solution of plasma prepared from the patient's own blood
- Platelets are alleged to release growth factors to enhance wound healing and have a rejuvenating effect
- This may be used in conjunction with other techniques such as laser resurfacing and microneedling (Box B)

5.9 **Question**

What is nanofat?

Answer

- Involves mechanically emulsifying harvested fat and filtering to a liquid suspension (Box C)
- Has been shown to improve scar quality in some initial papers
- Softening of scar tissue and a reduction in discoloration has been observed
- Nanofat enables injection more superficially than traditional fat grafts – a 27-gauge needle can be used, allowing better handling and versatility

---

Box A: Hypertrophic and keloid scars

- Hypertrophic scars usually occur within 8 weeks of injury and grow for up to 6 months
- They form in areas under tension and remain within the confines of the original wound
- Keloid scars also show no regression, extend beyond the original wound and frequently exhibit pain and hypersensitivity

---

Box B: Microneedling

- This is a minimally invasive procedure to create perforations to the level of the stratum corneum to increase skin permeability and stimulate growth factor release
- As the epidermal barrier is maintained, there is less risk of prolonged healing, infection, photosensitivity and pigmentation irregularities
- It can be used alone or in combination with topical agents or radiofrequency
- Automated devices such as the Dermapen are fixtures of nonsurgical cosmetic practice but have a role to play in traumatic scarring

---

Box C: Fat transfer

- Fat grafting can be used to address contour deformity
- Fat has inherent regenerative potential
- Lipoaspirate contains putative stem cells, endothelial cells and perivascular cells, sources of growth factors, cytokines, angiogenic factors and enzymes
- Fat is most commonly harvested from the abdomen using a 'wet' technique
- It can be harvested from redundant areas of the head and neck (e.g. submental supraplatysmal liposuction)
- Commonly aspiration is performed manually
- The lipoaspirate then centrifuged, but recent modifications have included power-assisted liposuction (e.g. PAL) and washing/filtration of fat (e.g. PureGraft system)

Further reading

Boahene KD, Owusu JA. Treating scars of the cheek region. Facial Plast Surg Clin North Am 2017; 25:37–43.

Fredman R, Katz AJ, Hultman CS. Fat grafting for burn, traumatic and surgical scars. Clin Plastic Surg 2017; 44:781–791.

Heffelfinger R, Sanan A, Bryant LM. Management of forehead scars. Facial Plast Surg Clin North Am 2017; 25:15–24.

Hivernaud V, Lefourn B, Robard M, et al. Autologous fat grafting: a comparative study of four current commercial protocols. J Plast Reconstr Aesthet Surg 2017; 70:248–256.

Long case 6: Dorsal nasal hump

The patient shown in the figure attends your aesthetic clinic wanting the hump on his nose improved.

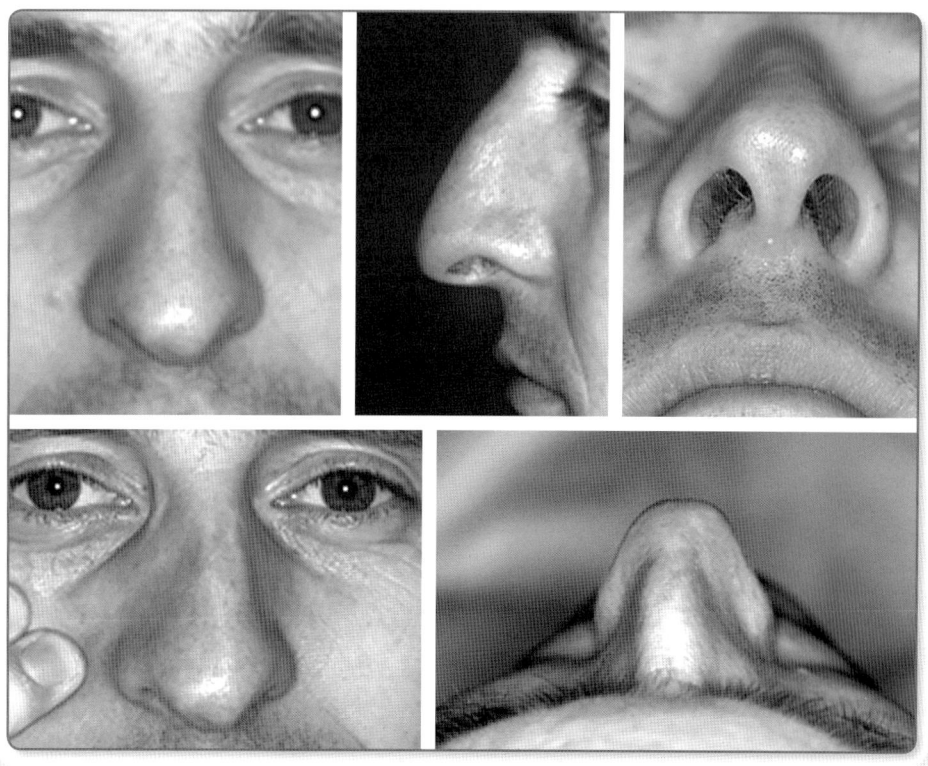

6.1 Question

What are the key features in the initial history?

Answer

- Determine key concerns: aesthetic, functional, both
- Ensure specificity about which exact components of nose are disliked
- Any problems breathing, snoring, during exercise
- Previous trauma/surgery
- Epistaxis
- Sinusitis/rhinitis/headaches
- Drug history: nasal decongestants, cocaine abuse
- Psychiatric: body dysmorphic disorder (BDD) and/or unrealistic expectations

6.2 Question

What are the key examination features?

Answer

Examine from front, lateral, worm's eye and bird's eye views (see figure):
- Relationship to rest of face: facial fifths
- Skin quality: thick/thin
- Symmetry/deviation
- Dorsal aesthetic lines
- Nasal tip: boxy/pinched/bulbous/ptotic (Box A)
- Nasal projection (Box B)
- Alar base width
- Nasofrontal angle
- Columella show
- Upper lip length
- Maxillary deficiency
- Evidence of previous surgery, e.g. transcolumellar scar, open roof deformity

6.3 Question

How would you assess airflow clinically?

Answer
- Open the internal valve to check for collapse with Cottle's test (see figure)
- Use Thudichum speculum
- Collapse of the internal valve
- Septal deviation/perforation
- Tumours/polyps
- Inferior turbinate hypertrophy

6.4 Question

What other investigations would you perform?

Answer
- A CT scan if there was evidence of previous trauma or concerns about pathology

6.5 Question

What types of rhinoplasty are available?

Answer
- Closed and open approaches
- Closed (endonasal): no external scars and faster recovery but more limited repertoire of correction
- Closed may be delivery or nondelivery, depending on whether or not the lower lateral cartilages are 'delivered' externally
- Open technique allows full visualisation and modification in situ
- Rhinoplasty (particularly secondary) commonly utilises grafts (Box C)

6.6 Question

What are the possible complications of rhinoplasty?

Answer

- Airway obstruction
- Epistaxis
- Septal haematoma and/or perforation
- Collapse due to insufficient septal support
- CSF rhinorrhea and/or meningitis
- Olfactory disturbance
- Dissatisfaction with residual deformity, particularly paying attention to:
  - Inverted 'V' deformity
  - Rocker deformity
  - Pollybeak deformity
  - Nasal valve collapse
  - Graft extrusion
  - Tip alteration (options to prevent this are shown in Box D)

Box A: Key terminology in describing nasal examination

- Tip-defining points: highest points of tip
- Nasal length: distance from radix to tip
- Tip projection: distance from nasal tip to alar-facial groove:
  - Supratip (breakpoint): just above domes of alar cartilage
  - Infratip: nasal tip to columella
  - Open roof deformity: dorsum after dorsal hump removal prior to infracturing lateral osteotomies
  - Soft triangle: Noncartilage area of nostril between rim and caudal border of alar cartilage
  - ULC: upper lateral cartilage
  - LLC: lower lateral (alar) cartilage

Box B: Nasal projection

- The 'ideal' nasolabial angle is 900–1050 in men and 950–1100 in women
- Nasal tip projection can be determined by:
  - Crumley method: projection:height:length = 3:4:5
  - Goode method: projection: length = 0.55:0.6
  - Simons method: projection = upper lip length

Box C: Types of cartilage graft

- Dorsal onlay grafts: used to augment nasal dorsum
- Spreader grafts: placed between dorsal septum and ULC to restore/maintain internal valve
- Columellar strut graft: placed between medial crura to maintain tip support +/- increase projection; combined with onlay as 'umbrella graft'
- Shield graft: adjacent to caudal edges of anterior middle crura to define tip
- Alar batten graft: placed in a pocket in the alar sidewall lateral to LLC to combat collapse of the external valve
- Alar spreader graft: spans lateral crura in between LLC and vestibular skin

Box D: Altering the nasal tip

- Resection of the alar cartilage, e.g. cephalic trim
- Cartilage grafts, e.g. shield grafts
- Suture techniques: transdomal sutures, interdomal sutures, medial crural fixation sutures and columella-septal sutures
- Depressor septi nasi division

Further reading

Gunter JP, Landecker A, Cochran CS. Frequently used grafts in rhinoplasty: nomenclature and analysis. Plast Reconstr Surg 2006; 118:14e–29e.
Park SS. Fundamental principles in aesthetic rhinoplasty. Clin Exp Otorhinolaryngol 2011; 4:55–66.
Rohrich RJ, Ahmad J. Rhinoplasty. Plast Reconstr Surg 2011; 128:49e–73e.